CPHRM Exam SECRETS

Study Guide
Your Key to Exam Success

CPHRM Test Review for the
Certified Professional in Healthcare
Risk Management Exam

Dear Future Exam Success Story:

Congratulations on your purchase of our study guide. Our goal in writing our study guide was to cover the content on the test, as well as provide insight into typical test taking mistakes and how to overcome them.

Standardized tests are a key component of being successful, which only increases the importance of doing well in the high-pressure high-stakes environment of test day. How well you do on this test will have a significant impact on your future, and we have the research and practical advice to help you execute on test day.

The product you're reading now is designed to exploit weaknesses in the test itself, and help you avoid the most common errors test takers frequently make.

How to use this study guide

We don't want to waste your time. Our study guide is fast-paced and fluff-free. We suggest going through it a number of times, as repetition is an important part of learning new information and concepts.

First, read through the study guide completely to get a feel for the content and organization. Read the general success strategies first, and then proceed to the content sections. Each tip has been carefully selected for its effectiveness.

Second, read through the study guide again, and take notes in the margins and highlight those sections where you may have a particular weakness.

Finally, bring the manual with you on test day and study it before the exam begins.

Your success is our success

We would be delighted to hear about your success. Send us an email and tell us your story. Thanks for your business and we wish you continued success.

Sincerely,

Mometrix Test Preparation Team

Need more help? Check out our flashcards at: http://MometrixFlashcards.com/CPHRM

Copyright © 2015 by Mometrix Media LLC. All rights reserved.
Written and edited by the Mometrix Exam Secrets Test Prep Team
Printed in the United States of America

TABLE OF CONTENTS

Top 20 Test Taking Tips 3
Clinical/Patient Safety 4
Risk Financing 16
Legal and Regulatory 24
Healthcare Operations 57
Claims and Litigation 82
Practice Test 85
    Practice Questions 85
    Answers and Explanations 93
Secret Key #1 - Time is Your Greatest Enemy 101
    Pace Yourself 101
Secret Key #2 - Guessing is not Guesswork 101
    Monkeys Take the Test 101
    $5 Challenge 102
Secret Key #3 - Practice Smarter, Not Harder 103
    Success Strategy 103
Secret Key #4 - Prepare, Don't Procrastinate 103
Secret Key #5 - Test Yourself 104
General Strategies 104
Special Report: How to Overcome Test Anxiety 110
    Lack of Preparation 110
    Physical Signals 111
    Nervousness 111
    Study Steps 113
    Helpful Techniques 114
Additional Bonus Material 119

Top 20 Test Taking Tips

1. Carefully follow all the test registration procedures
2. Know the test directions, duration, topics, question types, how many questions
3. Setup a flexible study schedule at least 3-4 weeks before test day
4. Study during the time of day you are most alert, relaxed, and stress free
5. Maximize your learning style; visual learner use visual study aids, auditory learner use auditory study aids
6. Focus on your weakest knowledge base
7. Find a study partner to review with and help clarify questions
8. Practice, practice, practice
9. Get a good night's sleep; don't try to cram the night before the test
10. Eat a well balanced meal
11. Know the exact physical location of the testing site; drive the route to the site prior to test day
12. Bring a set of ear plugs; the testing center could be noisy
13. Wear comfortable, loose fitting, layered clothing to the testing center; prepare for it to be either cold or hot during the test
14. Bring at least 2 current forms of ID to the testing center
15. Arrive to the test early; be prepared to wait and be patient
16. Eliminate the obviously wrong answer choices, then guess the first remaining choice
17. Pace yourself; don't rush, but keep working and move on if you get stuck
18. Maintain a positive attitude even if the test is going poorly
19. Keep your first answer unless you are positive it is wrong
20. Check your work, don't make a careless mistake

Clinical/Patient Safety

Human factors and patient safety

It is generally acknowledged that the majority of healthcare accidents are the result of human error. There are a number of disciplines that have emerged in an attempt to reduce these errors. They include ergonomics, human factors analysis, and human factors engineering. Ergonomics is the study of how people move and the effort to design equipment that will be easy to use properly. In the field of healthcare, ergonomics experts try to design spaces that are large enough for several employees to work without crowding one another. Human factors analysis requires a complete examination of the task, the employee, and the environment. The analyst takes into consideration the ratio of work to rest, the physical and mental abilities of the worker, and the noise and light in the surrounding area. Human factors engineering is the attempt to fit the equipment and environment to the size, strength, and coordination of the worker.

Systems thinking in relation to patient safety

In analyses of patient safety, experts often refer to systems thinking, by which they mean the interaction of many distinct factors. An emphasis on systems thinking is an acknowledgement that patient safety cannot be improved by isolating particular aspects of experience. Instead, a holistic approach is required. In healthcare, performance is based on an admixture of structural elements, inputs, outputs, and the physical environment of the facility. To understand the system, the analyst needs to know whether the elements exist in series, in parallel, or both. When systems are in parallel, one can fail without jeopardizing the other. One common exercise in systems thinking is the failure modes and effects analysis (FMEA), in which a team of experts tries to predict possible errors or breakdowns in the process before it is implemented.

Impact of hospital hierarchies on patient safety

In recent years, healthcare critics have noted that the traditional hierarchy of hospitals can contribute to errors. When a junior employee is concerned about the conduct of a senior employee or the condition of equipment, he or she typically voices this concern through the chain of command. However, there is an inevitable delay as information is passed up the hierarchy, and there are numerous opportunities for distortion or error. In the meantime, the behaviors or conditions about which the junior employee was complaining may have caused an adverse event. The problems associated with traditional complex hierarchies may be mitigated by devising a way for employees to register complaints immediately, and by generally simplifying the organizational hierarchy. Some healthcare facilities have addressed this problem with targeted programs, in which employees are encouraged to alert multiple superiors as soon as a risk is perceived.

SBAR

The situational briefing model (occasionally referred to as SBAR, for situation, background, assessment, and recommendation) is a system for improving better communication among healthcare providers. According to this model, there are certain steps that should be habitual for employees who notice a potential problem. First, before alerting a senior official, the employee should assess the patient and review the initial diagnosis. The employee should then ensure that he or she knows which physician to contact. Once these steps have been accomplished, the employee should follow the SBAR method: that is, he should communicate the situation, background, assessment, and recommendation. The summary of the situation should include the reporting employee's name, position, and department; the patient's name, condition, and location; and the suspected problem. The employee should include the following background details about the patient: initial diagnosis, date of admission, pertinent medical history, and brief summary of treatment to date. The employee should then provide an assessment, with attention to changes in any of the following: mental status, pain, respiration, blood pressure or pulse, skin color, wound drainage, bowel movements, and joint deformity. Finally, the employee should indicate his or her recommendation.

FMEA and root cause analysis

Failure modes and effects analysis (FMEA) is a preemptive system for reducing errors. Instead of waiting for a process to fail and then studying the failure, risk managers who employ FMEA brainstorm all of the ways in which a process could fail, and then develop methods to prevent or counteract these failures. For instance, when a facility introduces a new piece of equipment, it might conduct an FMEA of all the ways in which the equipment might fail. A root cause analysis, on the other hand, looks at the event after the accident has happened. Healthcare facilities that are accredited by the Joint Commission must complete a root cause analysis after every sentinel event. Moreover, accredited institutions are required to perform at least one comprehensive failure mode and effects analysis every year.

Models of systems failure and accident causation

One of the more popular models of systems failure with regard to medical errors was advanced by James Reason and is known as the "Swiss cheese model." In this model, major failures are the result of multiple small errors. Reason used the image of a series of slices of Swiss cheese, with the holes representing errors of various magnitudes. When the holes of several slices are aligned, a larger mistake may occur. Another important distinction in the study of medical error is between active and latent failures. An active failure is an action or decision that clearly leads to a larger mistake, while a latent failure is a condition or administrative policy that makes the larger mistake more likely. Scholars of accident causation also make use of the blunt end/sharp model, in which a distinction is made between administrative decisions (blunt end) and point-of-service actions (sharp end). The blunt end is responsible for collecting resources, but decisions made there may constrain the actions at the sharp end and contribute to employee errors.

Hindsight bias

Hindsight bias is the tendency to assign all blame for an accident to the person who most directly committed it. For instance, if an error is made during surgery, investigators tend to place all the blame on the surgeon instead of exploring the administrative decisions that may have set the stage for the error. This bias occurs because the investigator sees the situation from the perspective of the accident and its outcome, which tends to appear inevitable in hindsight. The resulting perception of the system failure is distorted. The practitioner who made the final error is assigned all the blame, and he or she may be punished or even fired without any attention being paid to the conditions that contributed to the accident.

Effects of lack of a common language

Many errors are the result of poor communication, and this in turn is often the result of the absence of a shared language. That is, medical practitioners may be unfamiliar with the various terminology and jargon that is so often used in the industry, and errors may be the result. As much as possible, the language used within a facility should be standardized. One effort to this end has been the creation of standard vocabularies for special subjects, as for instance the lexicon created by the National Institute of Child Health and Human Development with respect to fetal monitoring. The Joint Commission has also begun to encourage the use of checklists, readbacks, and site marking to reduce errors caused by poor communication.

Required information for prescriptions

Patient information
The first step in preventing medication errors is to ensure that sufficient patient information is acquired. The recording professional needs to be especially keen to record information related to allergies and comorbidities. However, the following pieces of patient information are all considered to be essential: renal and hepatic function; age, weight, and height; demographics; pregnancy and lactation status; medication history; lab results; diagnosis; and clinical observations. Of course, medical facilities must also observe strict protocols with respect to identifying information. The Joint Commission has mandated that practitioners use at least two patient-specific identifiers before administering medication; this policy drastically reduces instances of the wrong medication being delivered. Usually, the two pieces of identifying information are name and birth date. Patient identification data should always be compared to the medication administration record.

Drug information
The preponderance of medication errors occur because the most recent information about drugs is not present at the point of delivery. To minimize medication errors, the staff should be continually updated as to the uses, dosages, side effects, and interactions of medications. Many common medications have their usage protocols updated or altered, and employees should be kept abreast of these changes. The Joint Commission has recommended that practitioners only prescribe and administer those medications with which they are totally familiar. This means, of course, that facilities must allot time for staff to study. There are a few fledgling systems for making medication information available at the point of care. For instance, some healthcare facilities make use of computerized provider order entry (CPOE) systems, which present relevant information and results when medication is being ordered.

Drug labeling and packaging procedures

The appropriate procedures for drug labeling must be followed to avoid confusion. The Food and Drug Administration must approve the labels used by drug manufacturers, and in some cases it is necessary for the company to affix a sticker that clarifies any potential confusion while the labeling issue is being resolved. Whenever the medical staff perceives a risk of confusion, they should call attention to it with a pen or highlighter on the label. There are also bar coding systems that can minimize drug errors at the point of service. Errors can also arise because of confusing drug packaging, particularly when drugs have similar names or appearances. One way to reduce the confusion related to drug packaging is to use products from different manufacturers because each company has distinctive packaging. The risk of packaging errors can be exacerbated when medical staff discards the outer packaging before use. For instance, it is common practice in many facilities to remove all of a patient's medication from its packaging and place it in a cup. This practice improves efficiency but can increase the risk of medication being administered to the wrong patient. Again, bar coding at the point of service can mitigate this problem.

Reducing errors related to drug nomenclature

Medications often have long names, so practitioners can get into the habit of referring to them by abbreviations or nicknames. This can lead to errors. In addition, pharmaceutical manufacturers may introduce a new drug with a name similar to a popular drug already on the market. These problems can be addressed by insisting that the brand and generic names for each drug be included in the order, transcription, and prescription of all medication. One industry-wide strategy for reducing errors related to nomenclature is to use only the generic name for drugs with a single active ingredient. Perhaps the best defense against such errors, however, is common sense. Practitioners should be alert for situations in which the medication to be administered does not align with the patient's condition. In addition, both the generic and brand names should be listed on pharmacy labels and documentation.

Drug storage and stocking procedures

Errors are reduced when a medical facility has fewer locations for drug storage. In addition, facilities should put high-risk medications under lock and key, and should organize medications by function rather than alphabetically. Some facilities have attempted to solve the problem by installing automated dispensing devices, but when these are inefficient, employees may be more likely to store medication in their pockets. It is also imperative for the automated dispensing system to be integrated with the rest of the pharmacy's software. Employees should not be allowed to store high-risk drugs in their pockets. Moreover, drugs with a high risk of abuse should only be dispensed by the pharmacist.

Device acquisition and use procedures

The advent of human factors engineering has vastly improved the quality and reliability of the devices used to administer medication. In particular, infusion pumps have undergone radical changes in recent decades. This is especially important because infusion pump errors often have serious consequences for the patient. Despite the recent advances, however, infusion pumps are still susceptible to over-dosage errors. Some of the newest models include an electronic drug reference that will alert the user when an abnormally large amount of the drug is being administered. In particular, institutions should have a specific protocol for dealing with patient-controlled analgesia (PCA) pumps. These devices allow the patient to self-administer a very small dose of analgesia. While it is very difficult to overdose with a PCA pump, faulty pumps can lead to adverse effects.

Importance of patient monitoring to device maintenance

One of the most important ways for a practitioner to assess the performance of a medical device is to monitor the patient. The monitoring process should be based on a specific established protocol, which at the very least must include lab results, respiration, and vital signs. Many healthcare facilities have underscored the importance of monitoring by installing sophisticated computerized systems that keep track of staff performance. Healthcare professionals should have access to all of the important information related to the patient. Moreover, this information should be accessible from the patient's bedside. It may be necessary to stock specific medications or resuscitation equipment at the bedside. When this equipment is present, it should be indicated in the patient's paperwork. The ongoing records should include an assessment of the accuracy of previous monitoring efforts so that the medical facility can identify persistent biases or miscalculations.

Environmental stressors and medication errors

On occasion, medication errors can be the results of suboptimal environmental conditions in the facility. Indeed, the vast majority of transcription errors are the result of simple distraction. But as much as possible, medical staff should be able to prescribe, transcribe, prepare, and administer medications as part of a continuous process. In addition, facilities should discourage working conditions that contribute to employee fatigue. The number of medication errors dramatically increases when a nurse works more than 40 hours a week for 12 hours in a shift. For this reason, a medical facility needs to take specific steps to rest employees and ensure that staffing needs can be met without overburdening employees. In addition, medical practitioners should be prevented from engaging in any activities that could lead to distraction while handling medication.

Patient education and medication errors

Medication errors are significantly reduced when patients are alert and informed. Patients should be told the standard procedures prior to administration, as well as the general schedule for medication. Detailed information related to drug selection, indications, typical doses, possible drug or food interactions, and possible side effects should be made available to patients. Moreover, patients should be encouraged to ask questions and seek more detailed information. Medical staff should not assume a high level of medical literacy among the general patient population. Many patients will need direct explanation from trained staff. In some cases, it may be necessary to enlist the participation of a specific professional, as for instance a pharmacist or surgeon.

Prioritizing approaches to manage risks of medication errors

In order to implement a successful program for diminishing medical errors, a risk management professional needs to prioritize the related interventions and issues. In other words, the risk management professional should place the most emphasis on those strategies that will produce the greatest results. In general, error reduction strategies can be grouped from most to least important as follows: forcing functions and constraints, automation and computerization, standardization and protocols, checklists and double check systems, rules and policies, and education and information. Forcing functions and constraints are decisions and using products that do not allow for the possibility of error. It is only slightly less effective to automate or computerize processes: there is still a small risk of malfunction, but it is drastically reduced. Medical professionals should also be aware of the riskiest patients and procedures. The patients with the highest risk of medication error are oncology patients, newborns, the elderly, pregnant women, patients with renal or liver damage, or patients taking several medications. The processes most often involved in medication error are patient-controlled analgesia, epidural analgesia, allergy testing, and preparation of mixed medications using automated compounders.

Communication protocols to minimize medication errors

There are certain communication protocols that can minimize medication errors. Communication problems in this context can be much more complex than mishearing or misunderstanding an order. For example, many hospitals have drug information systems that cannot communicate with the laboratory system or the electronic medical record system. When this is the case, it is inevitable that medication errors will be made. When the facility does not have a computerized provider order entry system, there is a much greater risk of errors caused by bad handwriting or unclear commands. More abstractly, dysfunctional relationships between staff members can result in medication errors. In many healthcare facilities, subordinates do not feel comfortable challenging or questioning orders from their superiors, and so clear errors go uncorrected. Many facilities are attempting to minimize these problems by eliminating spoken orders and devising a standard protocol for written orders.

Medication error reporting and follow-up

In order for a medication error reporting system to be effective, employees must feel empowered to report errors when they occur. Moreover, employees need to feel confident that incident reports will lead to improvements in the delivery system. Essentially, risk managers need to incentivize reporting. Employees who report errors should not be subject to unnecessary scrutiny or investigation. The risk manager is responsible for establishing this culture of communication. For instance, the risk manager should ensure that the focus of discussion related to medication errors is improving the patient experience, not punishing those who committed the errors.

Problems with patient-controlled analgesia

PCA by proxy
One of the more common problems with patient-controlled analgesia (PCA) occurs when a person besides the patient administers the medication. This is known as PCA by proxy, and it is dangerous because the medication can be administered even after the patient has become sedated. (Normally, the patient loses consciousness before he or she can overdose.) PCA by proxy has been associated with respiratory depression, over-sedation, and (in rare cases) death. Medical facilities should make the dangers of PCA proxy known to both employees and visitors. Stickers warning of the risk of PCA by proxy should be attached to the activation buttons. In addition, medical facilities should keep PCA flow sheets by the side of the patient's bed. These flow sheets should be used to monitor the patient's condition and record PCA doses.

Improper patient selection and education
Not every patient in need of analgesia is a candidate for patient-controlled analgesia devices. These devices should only be used with patients who have demonstrated the

mental and physical competence. Many practitioners think of PCA pump-related errors only in terms of over-dosage, but if the patient is not strong or alert enough to administer enough of the medication, the device must be considered a failure as well. Patients should not be instructed as to the use of the PCA pump immediately after surgery or sedation. Hospitals must use some basic test of alertness to determine if the patient is competent to understand the instructions. It is always best to describe the use of the PCA pump to the patient before the operation. The hospital should also apply strict limitations on the patients who are allowed to use a PCA pump. Most facilities do not allow infants, small children, or mentally unstable patients to use these devices. In addition, the hospital staff should ensure that the patient does not have any allergies that could complicate the use of a PCA pump.

Insufficient patient monitoring

When patients are not monitored sufficiently, there is a risk of error in the use of patient-controlled analgesia (PCA) pumps. A simple physical response test is not always enough to ascertain the patient's level of consciousness. Similarly, staff should not rely on pulse oximetry by itself; even when respiration is very low, oxygen saturation rates may remain normal. To guard against errors caused by insufficient monitoring, nurses should be well schooled in observing the signs and symptoms of opiate toxicity. The facilities should establish a standard scale for pain assessment, and should have an assessment protocol that minimizes verbal or tactile stimulation. When a patient is using a PCA pump, his or her vital signs (including respiration) should be assessed at least every four hours. Moreover, the patient should be monitored more often in the 24 hours following surgery, as well as at night (because of the greater risk of nocturnal hypoxia or hypoventilation). Both oxygen and naloxone should be stationed by the bedside of the patient.

Medication confusion

Like many other medications, patient-controlled analgesics are subject to errors caused by confusing labeling or packaging. In particular, morphine and meperidine have often been confused because they are packaged in similar containers. Also, a number of patients have overdosed after staff used the floor stock of opiates (which is typically much stronger) in patient-controlled analgesia (PCA) pumps. To safeguard against medication confusion, facilities should place clear warning labels on any nonstandard concentrations, and should generally stick to one standard concentration for all of the opiates used in PCAs. Hydromorphone and morphine are often confused, so they should be stored separately. Whenever possible, facilities should use syringes, bags, and cassettes that are prefilled by the manufacturer. Before any PCA orders are initiated, the pharmacy should conduct a basic review of the prescription. Staff should be required to conduct independent double checks of patient identification, administered drug (including concentration), pump settings, and line attachment. Finally, clinicians should be warned about any drug shortages, and the facility should have an established protocol for alternative dosing.

Improper programming of the PCA pump and errors of dosage

Most patient-controlled analgesia (PCA) errors occur because the pump is programmed incorrectly. These errors can be minimized, however, by using the same pump model throughout the facility. Also, a set of laminated instructions should be affixed to each pump. The newer pumps can be programmed to require a confirmation of the settings before delivery. The facility should also take steps to reduce errors caused by incorrect transcription, IV admixture, and the miscalculation of rate of infusion or dose. The likelihood of these errors can be diminished by requiring independent double checks of administered drug, dosage, concentration, pump settings, line attachment, and patient identification.

Errors in device design
Some patient-controlled analgesia (PCA) errors can be attributed to flaws in the design of the device. For instance, on some devices it is difficult to distinguish the infusion button with the nurse call button, which can lead to overdosing or underdosing. Other devices have default settings, which are usually set low, but may still dispense a higher concentration of the medicine. In some cases, a broken cassette or syringe will go unnoticed because of automatic programming. There are a few ways to mitigate this sort of error. One is to set the default for all opiates at zero. Another is to ensure that the PCA pump is connected to a port close to the patient: this will decrease the chances of the infusion line becoming confused. In most medical facilities, pumps are programmed to alert staff and stop infusion if the syringe or bag becomes damaged. Errors related to the device design will also be diminished when a single model of PCA pump is used. Finally, it should be mandated that pumps are programmed in milligrams per milliliter and micrograms per milliliter, as well as simply in milliliters.

Insufficient training of staff
Problems with patient-controlled analgesia (PCA) can arise when staff are poorly trained, or when their training is not refreshed regularly. These problems are especially common when several different types of pumps are used, or when PCA pumps are not used very often. To prevent errors caused by poor training, medical facilities should standardize PCA training and subject it to periodic review. In addition, staff members should be required to pass an annual competency test. Whenever PCA pumps are used, the facility should require independent double checks of the pump settings, line attachment, administered drug, concentration, and patient identification. If possible, the facility should only use a single model of PCA pump. Also, a set of laminated instructions should be affixed to each pump.

Errors in communication of orders
Dangerous errors may occur when a patient who has been receiving oral opiates begins to receive his or her medication through an IV. Hydromorphone is the drug most often involved in this sort of error. In some cases, medication becomes confused because a patient-controlled analgesia (PCA) pump is already in use as other opiate orders are made. The result can be opiate toxicity. To prevent this type of error, many medical facilities implement standard order sets, including necessary precautions, doses, lockout periods, and drug selection. Also, some facilities restrict verbal orders to dose changes. A facility should also require independent double checks of patient identification, administered drug, concentration, pump settings, and line attachment. Most facilities also apply general rules to their use of opiates. For instance, in a typical arrangement the facility will use morphine as the normal medication, hydromorphone when unusually high doses are needed, and meperidine for patients who are allergic to morphine and hydromorphone.

Early identification of loss exposures

In order for a risk management program to do its job, the organization must be able to identify loss exposures before they result in liability. The risk manager needs to have early warning systems in place to identify any potentially compensable events, adverse events, systems errors, claims, and near misses. The risk manager must not limit his or her evaluation to clinical or operational risks because the organization is potentially liable for all of its actions, not just those relating to the provision of health services. It is very important for a risk manager to develop a culture of communication, and even whistleblowing, so that the staff becomes the first line of defense against liability.

Identifying early warnings of risk

There are a few basic procedures for identifying the early warnings of risk. Most organizations employ what is known as enterprise risk management, in which the potential for loss is evaluated throughout the entire organization. To begin with, the risk manager will make a list of all of the risks intrinsic to the operations of the organization, regardless of its specific methodologies. The risk manager will want to pay particular attention to the relationships between risks and the ways in which risks may combine with and even magnify one another. As an example, the risk manager might consider the ways in which maintaining a smaller staff could increase the likelihood of errors. The risk manager will also need to identify the patterns of communication and the hierarchies within the organization, as these may create the possibility of loss or may suggest strategies for minimizing risk.

Handling disruptive patients or family members

The Joint Commission has outlined some specific recommendations for how the staff of a medical facility should handle disruptive patients or family members. To begin with, the Joint Commission suggests that facilities should have a clear definition of disruptive or inappropriate behavior, and that this definition be known by staff. In addition, the facility should make staff responsible for modeling appropriate behavior, and should give positive reinforcement to those members of the staff who meet expectations. There must be some sort of surveillance program in place so that the administrators of the facility can monitor the behavior of patients and staff. When interventions are necessary to respond to disruptive behavior, the staff should be sure to listen to and express empathy with the concerns of the patient, but should reiterate the protocols and discuss the consequences of disruptive behavior.

Medical error reporting requirements

The Joint Commission, as well as various state and federal bodies, have mandated that healthcare facilities report certain incidents immediately. For instance, the Sentinel Event Policy of the Joint Commission declares that the following events must be reported: abduction of a patient, rape, discharge of an infant to the wrong family, hemolytic transfusion reaction, improper surgery, severe neonatal hyperbilirubinemia, unintended retention of a foreign object inside a patient, and prolonged fluoroscopy with a cumulative dose greater than 1500 rads to a single field. There are similar adverse event reporting systems in 26 states. A risk manager must be familiar with these programs, as well as with the federal reporting requirements associated with legislation like the Safe Medical Devices Act.

Formal internal reporting methods

Every healthcare organization should have in place several formal internal reporting methods, or procedures for identifying risk. Indeed, the insurance companies typically require healthcare providers to implement these systems as a prerequisite for coverage.

There are also formal internal reporting methods established and promoted by the National Committee for Quality Assurance, the Commission for Accreditation of Rehabilitation Facilities, the Utilization Review Accreditation Committee, and the Joint Commission. Some facilities may be subject to the requirements of state statutes as well. These reporting methods are described as internal because they are meant to be used for communication between members of the same organization.

Incident reports

The standard incident report was developed by commercial insurance companies for recording events, claims, and losses. These companies find it useful to be notified by policyholders whenever an event has occurred that may result in a claim. The most basic version of the form includes information about the patient and the incident. Healthcare organizations have come to find these documents so useful that they are often maintained even when not required by an insurance carrier. In the context of this form of reporting, an incident is defined as any event that is inconsistent with routine care or operations. Many organizations employ electronic incident reporting systems so that the data can be easily analyzed. Indeed, a number of risk management information systems are available at present, many of them designed for specific types of institution.

Essential contents
An incident report must include certain basic information in order for it to be useful to the risk management department. To begin with, these reports should include some demographic information about the patient, including name, address, telephone number, and medical record number. An incident report should also include essential information about the facility, as for instance the patient's admission or visit date, the business number associated with the incident, the patient room number, and the reason for the visit. The incident report should include some basic socioeconomic data about the patient, including his or her age, gender, marital status, occupation, and insurance status. The incident report should contain a brief description of the incident, including where it occurred, the type of incident, the degree to which the patient was injured, and the results of any post-incident examination.

Common obstacles to incident reporting
It is essential for the risk manager to promote communication among staff members. Some of the common obstacles to incident reporting are a lack of clear protocols for reporting, or a perception that whistleblowers will be punished, either directly or implicitly. In some facilities, staff members are overworked and fail to complete incident reports because they do not have enough time. Incident reporting may also be discouraged in institutions where there is a clear class distinction between physicians and non-physicians; it may be that non-physicians are too intimidated to report instances in which the physician may be culpable. If the facility does not do a good job of maintaining confidentiality standards, then the result may be an unwillingness to report incidents.

Confidentiality
Confidentiality is particularly important with respect to incident reports because a perception that reports will not be kept confidential may discourage employees from reporting incidents in the future. Every state has legislation guaranteeing the confidentiality of these reports. After the incident report has been drafted, it should be sent directly to the risk manager. The risk manager should never make copies of the report, and should never

include it in the medical record. Whenever other professionals need to review incident reports, as for instance during quality improvement tasks, this should always be done inside the risk manager's office, and the originals should not be copied or allowed to leave the care of the risk manager. It should be noted that, while incident report confidentiality is protected by the law, these documents can be examined as part of the discovery process before a trial. For this reason, incident reports should be limited to matters of fact, and should avoid speculation or conjecture.

Occurrence reporting

Occurrences related to surgery, treatment, procedures, blood, intravenous treatment, and medication-related occurrences must be reported. Blood-related occurrences include delivery of the wrong type of blood, transmission of disease through infected blood, and the improper use of blood products. Treatment and procedure occurrences include excessive exposure to X-rays, burns caused by hot packs, and adverse reactions to the contrast material used in a diagnostic procedure. Surgery occurrences include operations on the wrong patient or site, the use of the wrong procedure, or an incorrect sponge or instrument count. Intravenous occurrences include the administration of the wrong solution, an incorrect infusion rate, or the infiltration of solution. The most common medication-related claims are for the wrong dosage, route, frequency, choice of medication, medication used, time, administration technique, patient, or reason for medication. Medication-related claims may also be related to a missed dose, a known drug interaction, or a known drug allergy. Occurrence reports must also be filed when there is a lack of adequate follow-up or when a patient falls.

<u>Emergency department occurrence reporting criteria</u>
Emergency departments are required to file a report when any patient leaves against medical advice or without being seen. A report is required for patients who make an unscheduled return to the emergency room within 72 hours. The emergency department must also file reports after patient falls, medication errors, incidents of assault or violence, missing or inadequate discharge instructions, or any failures to diagnose a condition. Reports must also be filed after any failure to use or deliver thrombolytics or initiate treatment in a timely manner. Whenever a patient is misidentified or there is an ineffective hand-off to another part of the facility, a report must be filed. Finally, a report is required after any failure to remove a foreign body or after inadequate medication reconciliation.

Occurrence screening

The occurrence screening system is a standardized method for identifying adverse patient events. Like many other observation systems, it establishes a baseline for practice, and then seeks to identify deviations from this baseline. The particular criteria depend on the type of facility. Although occurrence screening is primarily used in acute care facilities, it may also be applied in ambulatory care facilities, medical clinics, and physician group practices. A proper occurrence screening system requires the work of trained data retrieval employees who look over the number of events and analyze them. Because this system relies heavily on a department of specially-trained personnel, it is important for the risk manager to be proactive about staying involved and informed. The risk manager should review the data analyses and be alert to trends in occurrences.

Improving the reporting process

There are a few strategies that can be used to improve the reporting process. For instance, a risk manager might take a look at committee meeting minutes, in particular those related to patient safety, bioethics, and quality assurance. The risk manager might also examine claims data, survey reports, patient complaints, and standardized patient satisfaction surveys. Some of the best survey reports are those created by the Joint Commission, Occupational Safety and Health Administration, Commission on Accreditation of Rehabilitation Facilities, and National Commission on Accreditation of Rehabilitation Facilities. The risk manager should make sure that the list of reportable occurrences is created through a collaboration of doctors and senior managers. The risk manager should try to minimize the paperwork associated with incident reporting, and should return the results of the incident review to the appropriate departments as quickly as possible, while the incident remains fresh in the minds of the relevant employees.

Risk Financing

Risk retention strategies

Sometimes, a risk manager determines that it makes more sense to settle claims related to certain risks as they occur than to acquire insurance against these losses. This is known as risk retention. The four major strategies of risk retention are the use of operating funds, the creation of loss reserves, the use of borrowed funds, and self-insurance. The use of operating funds is the most casual approach. This is a typical strategy for paying the deductibles on property losses. Of course, this is not a good strategy for handling large losses that occur unexpectedly. For these, an institution may want to create loss reserves, the sizes of which are based on actuarial assessment of the likelihood and severity of the loss. For some large institutions, it may make sense to borrow funds when losses occur. However, small facilities usually avoid this strategy because it reduces the ability to borrow money for other purposes. Finally, healthcare facilities may retain risk by ensuring themselves, usually either through a self-insurance trust or a captive insurance company.

Risk retention and risk transfer

There are a number of factors that will influence the decision of whether to retain or transfer risk. To begin with, the risk manager should consider the size and structure of the organization, as well as the financial strength of the ownership. The risk manager will also need to consider the type of risk, and the potential consequences of failing to manage it. The risk manager will need to take into account the risk philosophy of the organization, and the recent success of the risk management and loss control programs. Finally, the risk manager should consider the goals and objectives of the organization and whether the accomplishment of these will be influenced by the selection of risk management strategies. Some medical facilities prefer to use risk financing strategies because these provide a mixture of risk transfer and risk retention.

Formal self-insurance techniques

The two primary formal self-insurance techniques are the self-insurance trust and the captive insurance company. A self-insurance trust is a bank account run by a third party, known as the trustee. The funds contained in a self-insurance trust are specifically designated for paying losses. The schedule of payments to the trust is based on an actuarial study. A trust is not defined as an insurance vehicle, so it cannot pay for any losses other than those for which it was created. It is more common at present for healthcare facilities to self-insure by means of a captive insurance company, which is to say an insurance company primarily funded and operated by its owners, and in which the principal beneficiaries are the original insureds. A captive insurance company is essentially created for the sole purpose of handling the healthcare facilities loss. The advantages of a captive insurance policy are that it may be structured in a way that is beneficial to the finances of the healthcare facility.

Strategies for risk transfer

In a risk transfer agreement, the losses incurred by the healthcare facility are paid for by a third party. A commercial insurance policy is the most obvious form of risk transfer, although it is also possible to transfer risk through an indemnification contract provision. Purchasing commercial insurance is, at its essence, the transfer of risk to the insurance company. To an extent, the healthcare facility retains part of the risk, insofar as a deductible must be paid. In an indemnification provision, on the other hand, two parties agree that when one party sufferers liability, loss, or damage, the other party will make any necessary payments. These provisions are sometimes called hold harmless agreements. The indemnification agreement makes sense for supply or construction contracts, but it is rarely used with respect to professional services. A patient, for instance, would probably decline to sign a hold harmless agreement with his or her physician in advance of treatment.

Insurance

Insurance policies protect their owners from the risk of loss. In exchange for a regular payment, the policy holder receives compensation if the insured property is damaged or destroyed, or if an insured person is injured or killed. The following are common policy conditions: the obligation of the insured to pay the premium in a timely manner; the conditions under which the policy may be canceled or under which renewal may be denied; the obligation of the insured to give prompt notice of loss; the obligation of the insured to assist the insurer in the investigation and settlement of a loss; the right of the insured to inspect the premises; the policy's coverage territory; and the applicability of deductibles, limits, and defense expenses. An exclusion is a policy provision that diminishes or eliminates coverage. Some of the more common exclusions are intentional acts, war, criminal conduct, mold, and nuclear energy.

Insurance regulation

For the most part, insurance regulation is handled by the states. Every insurance broker or agent must be licensed in each state in which he or she operates. Typically, obtaining licensure requires passing a state examination and fulfilling continuing education requirements. Insurance carriers that have been approved (also known as admitted insurers) must submit all current policy forms, changes in forms, and premium rate increases or decreases to the state insurance department. A company may elect to operate as a non-admitted or surplus line carrier, and therefore be exempt from state regulations. However, surplus line carriers are not allowed to participate in the guaranty fund, which means that policyholders are required to pay taxes or other fees in addition to the normal premium.

Evaluating the financial status of insurance companies

Before deciding to transfer risk, a risk manager should take a close look at the financial status of the insurance carrier. There are limited sources of compensation for organizations that have policies with failed carriers. When a state guaranty fund only provides partial compensation, the insured organization will be responsible for the difference. There are a number of insurance carrier rating organizations, the most acclaimed of which is A.M. Best Co., which issues a rating from "A++" to "F" based on the carrier's profitability, leverage, capitalization, and liquidity. These evaluations are objectively derived from the carrier's spread of risk exposures, diversification of assets, capital structure, adequacy of surplus and loss reserves, policyholders' confidence, and market presence.

Purchasing insurance

When purchasing commercial insurance policies, a healthcare risk manager typically operates through an agent or broker. A broker is an independent insurance professional who is adept at assessing risk potential, gathering information related to exposure and loss, negotiating coverage terms and the price of premiums, and evaluating quotes from insurance companies. In some cases, insurance brokers are also able to assist in the mitigation of losses, and even to come up with alternative means of risk financing. Brokers typically represent the interests of the insurance carrier, and are compensated on a commission basis. Many brokers accept a flat fee, which eliminates the incentive to sell the customer more insurance then he or she needs. In any case, the broker is required to disclose his or her compensation upon the request of the customer.

Drafting coverage specifications

Risk managers need to be entirely certain that they are acquiring sufficient but not excessive insurance coverage for their institutions. It is usual for the first step to be the composition of an underwriting submission, which is a summary of the required insurance. A typical underwriting submission contains the following elements: description of operations; organizational chart; list of named insured parties and additional insureds; retroactive dates; large loss detail; current annual report and any other relevant financial statements; signed application; accreditation report (usually from the Joint Commission); location listing; current and historical exposure information; trust, captive, or underlying coverage document; large loss detail for any claim over $100,000; currently valued historical loss experience; summary of risk management policies; and a description of the limits, deductibles, coverages, and policy period.

Selecting an insurance carrier

Selecting an insurance carrier is one of the most important decisions a risk manager will make. To begin with, the risk manager needs to ensure that policy is aligned with the short- and long-term goals of the healthcare institution. The risk manager should also evaluate the financial standing of the insurance carrier, specifically by evaluating its rating by A.M. Best or another such organization. The risk manager should also consider whether the insurance carrier is familiar with healthcare operations, and whether it is flexible enough to accommodate the changing needs of such an institution. The risk manager should consider the pricing system, and the extent to which future prices will be influenced by events in the healthcare industry. The risk manager may also want to consider how long the insurance carrier has been offering this particular type of coverage, and whether its performance has been acceptable in the past. Finally, the risk manager should take a look at the carrier's procedures for handling claims.

Hard and soft insurance markets

In a hard insurance market, a risk manager should take into account the carrier's approach to business, as well as its historic involvement in the healthcare industry. The risk manager will want to consider the approach taken by the carrier during previous pricing cycles. The risk manager should evaluate the financial status of the business and the loss ratio it has had with similar policies. It may be sensible to distribute the exposures to several carriers, although often an institution can receive some sort of discount when it places all of its business with the same carrier. A soft market, on the other hand, exists when the pricing and terms of insurance policies are relatively flexible. When the market is considered to be soft, it may be advisable for the institution to renegotiate its insurance coverage.

Amount of insurance to purchase and limits of liability

It can be difficult to decide how much insurance to purchase. A risk manager must rely on the purchase history, the legal climate, and the regulatory environment. The risk manager may also want to compare the insurance coverages obtained by similar facilities. The risk manager will also want to consider the amount of risk being retained by self-insurance or a deductible, as well as the limits to be obtained. The risk manager will also need to consider the limits of liability, or the maximum amount of compensation that may be provided by the insurer. The limits of liability may be defined as an annual aggregate or per occurrence. Some policies also contain sublimits, which is a cap on the amount that a policy will pay for one particular peril. The sublimit is not an addition to the policy limit.

Named peril and all-risk coverage

Medical facilities may purchase either named peril or all-risk coverage to protect themselves against direct damage losses. Most facilities select all-risk coverage because it applies to a broader range of losses. Indeed, all-risk policies only exclude those events that are specifically mentioned. Some of the perils that are typically excluded from all-risk policies are intentional loss, normal wear and tear, earthquake, landslide, flood, and certain business risks. If a business has a particularly great exposure to one of these risks, it may be possible to obtain limited coverage for a slightly higher rate. Moreover, with an all-risk policy the burden of proof for demonstrating that a loss should not be covered lies with the insurance company. With a named peril policy, on the other hand, the only covered losses are those mentioned by name in the policy, and the insured party is responsible for proving that there has been a loss.

Time element coverage

Time element insurance coverage protects a business against a loss of revenue caused by an insured loss. In other words, whereas direct damage coverage provides compensation for the specific cause of the loss, time element coverage provides compensation for the revenue lost while the business recovers from that loss. The most common form of time element coverage is business interruption, which covers ordinary payroll and the extra expenses required to keep the facility running during the repair process. It can be quite difficult for the insurance company to adjust time element claims because the calculation of lost revenue can be very complex. One way that insurance carriers try to resolve this problem is by completing a business interruption worksheet every year, on which the insured party indicates the loss of income and continuing expenses that would be incurred by a partial or total closure of the facility.

Insurance coverage for electronic data processing and media

Many healthcare facilities must acquire insurance coverage for electronic data processing and media, which, unlike other pieces of equipment, may be damaged by dust and relatively minor changes in temperature and humidity. If this equipment or material is damaged, the business could be significantly interrupted for a long time. The business may find it is a good idea to purchase insurance that covers the cost of time-sharing facilities and equipment rental. These policies also often cover extra payroll expenses and temporary employees. Businesses may opt for a separate electronic data processing policy or an extension on their standard property policy. A typical electronic data processing policy will cover the expense of replacing any information lost from a card, drum, tape, or disk.

Insurance coverage for commercial crime and employee dishonesty

Many healthcare facilities, especially those with many employees, acquire commercial crime insurance as a hedge against losses due to crime committed by employees and others. These losses are not covered by the standard property insurance policies; commercial crime insurance covers losses from theft, robbery, disappearance, destruction, burglary, and employee dishonesty. There are also special policies that provide extra coverage against loss caused by employee dishonesty. These policies generally cover losses caused by the alteration of financial records or the theft of inventory. For medical facilities, these losses may be related to the theft of medication or other supplies. Computer crime by employees is an increasing problem, and many of the most recent commercial crime policies include provisions specifically related to this problem.

Third-party insurance

A third-party insurance policy covers the insured against any injury, damage, or loss caused by the negligence of the insured. It is called third-party insurance because the insurer, the insured, and the injured party are all involved. The most common third-party liability coverages for healthcare organizations are automobile, umbrella excess, medical professional, general (i.e., premises, independent contractor, contractual, personal injury), directors' and officers', miscellaneous errors and omissions, environmental impairment, and fiduciary. Third-party insurance is distinct from first-party insurance in that the named insured is never compensated directly for the loss or damage. Instead, the payment goes to the owner of the property damaged or destroyed by the named insured.

Insurance coverage for medical professional liability

Healthcare institutions acquire medical professional liability insurance to cover claims related to improper or incomplete delivery of medical services. This insurance may also cover damage related to medication, the handling of bodies after death, and the actions of formal professional boards and accreditation committees. In most medical facilities, professionals are required to maintain their own individual medical professional liability coverage. The most recent versions of this type of policy should include the following coverage: contractual liability; miscellaneous errors and omissions; utilization management and review; confidentiality; architects' or builders' legal liability; Medicare billing errors, fraud, and abuse; marketing; antitrust or restraint of trade; and third-party claims administration. Medical professional liability insurance policies are offered on the claims-made or the occurrence basis.

Insurance coverage for commercial general liability

A commercial general liability policy protects the healthcare institution against liability for losses unrelated to the performance of medical service. For instance, a commercial general liability policy would cover losses related to the premises or to products that originated on the premises. It also would cover the actions of independent contractors hired by the institution. A commercial general liability policy typically covers person injury allegations, property damage, and bodily injury, and most often is provided by the same insurance company that provides the facility with medical professional liability coverage. Indeed, these two forms of coverage are often components of the same policy. It is important for the risk manager to understand the various ways in which his or her facility could become liable for problems unrelated to medical services, and to ensure that these losses are covered by the commercial general liability policy.

Managed care errors and omissions insurance coverage

Managed care errors and omissions (E&O) insurance coverage have become more common with the rise of this type of health institution. Managed care institutions include HMOs, independent practice associations, management service organizations, physician-hospital organizations, and preferred provider organizations. A managed care E&O policy protects the institution against claims resulting from negligence or mistakes in the design and implementation of a managed care plan. The following are the most common negligence allegations against managed care organizations: discrimination, improper design or administration of cost control systems, breach of patient confidentiality, violations of the Employee Retirement Income Security Act of 1974, physician incentive agreements, antitrust, economic credentialing, violations of state insurance regulations, denial of benefits or service, bankruptcy, insolvency, and invasion of privacy.

Excess umbrella liability insurance

Medical institutions are uniquely susceptible to catastrophic loss, which can endanger the long-term survival of the organization. For this reason, many institutions obtain excess umbrella liability coverage, which provides compensation after the primary layer of liability coverage has been used up. An excess umbrella liability policy can be drafted to include medical professional liability, employer's liability, commercial general liability, automobile liability, and many other policies. It is essential for the primary and excess policies to have the same effective date, and for those dates to be written on concurrent coverage forms. When the primary layer of insurance is on a claims-made basis, the excess coverage should be written on that basis as well. If the primary coverage is written on an occurrence basis and the excess coverage is written on a claims-made basis, two sets of loss data will need to be compiled by the risk manager.

Automobile liability insurance

Most healthcare facilities maintain a fleet of owned, leased, or hired automobiles. Moreover, many of these facilities maintain parking garages, which create another area of significant loss exposure. A standard commercial automobile policy will cover any loss related to the ownership, maintenance, or use of cars. To cover automobiles not owned by the company, excess insurance will be required. Most standard automobile liability policies include personal injury protection and uninsured motorists' coverage. The cost of automobile coverage will depend on the territory within which the vehicles are used, the loss history, the type of vehicle, and the manner in which the vehicle is used. Most insurance providers require healthcare employees to undergo training in safe driving at least every two years as a condition of coverage.

Directors' and officers' liability insurance

Because the directors and officers of a healthcare facility are required to make important decisions, they often obtain specific insurance coverage against losses caused by these decisions. The intention of directors' and officers' (D&O) liability insurance is to forestall personal liability litigation against executives. One of the areas in which this sort of litigation is increasing is medical staff decision-making. Many facilities obtain D&O insurance against suits related to the hiring, promotion, or termination of employees. In particular, executives have been subject to antitrust lawsuits alleging that they have restrained trade by favoring one group of employees or by denying employment to a particular class of prospective employee. D&O insurance can also protect executives from liability related to mergers, acquisitions, and divestiture activities.

Employment practices and fiduciary liability insurance

Employment practices liability insurance may be purchased separately, though it is often included as part of a directors' and officers' liability policy. Employment practices liability insurance covers liability related to negligence in employment issues, as for instance selection and hiring. The advances in anti-discrimination rules, while positive in the aggregate, have increased the chances of liability for healthcare institutions. For instance, institutions may accidentally run afoul of the Americans with Disabilities Act. Fiduciary liability insurance, on the other hand, has been shaped in large part by the Employee Retirement Income Security Act of 1974 (ERISA). Any institution with more than 25 employees is subject to ERISA, and therefore should obtain insurance for those executives who are responsible for employee benefit plans. These policies protect against allegations of negligence or breach of fiduciary responsibility.

Employee benefit legal insurance and environmental impairment liability insurance

Employee benefit legal insurance protects the administrators of employee benefit plans from liability related to the administration of employee benefit plans. These policies cover all of the risks unrelated to regulations of the Employee Retirement Income Security Act of 1974, as for instance Social Security, unemployment compensation, workers compensation, and mandatory non-occupational disability benefit programs. Environmental impairment liability insurance, on the other hand, protects facilities from liability related to contaminated properties. The law defines environmental impairment as the propagation or spread of dangerous substances through soil, air, or water. These substances may include radiation, gases, heat, pressure, or noise. These policies are important because they cover gradual contamination, whereas most commercial general liability policies only cover sudden and accidental contamination.

Employee benefit insurance and workers' compensation insurance

Employee benefit insurance protects the administrators of employee benefit plans. In most cases, these plans are administered by the human resources department, but on occasion the risk manager will be called in to oversee or review the process. Because employee benefit plans may include life, vision, long- and short-term disability, accident, dental, and health insurance, a risk manager should be familiar with all of these coverages. Workers' compensation insurance is necessary in every state because every state requires employers to compensate employees who are injured during the course of their employment. Workers' compensation insurance is a classic example of no-fault insurance. The sources of employer's liability claims are injuries not covered by the act, employees who reject the act, suits by a spouse for loss of consortium or companionship, or a suit by a third party that has been held liable for the injury and seeks reimbursement from the employer.

Surety bonds and provider stop-loss coverage

Surety bonds are an arrangement in which two parties agree to pay damages to a third party if the principal (one of the original two parties) cannot meet an agreed-upon financial obligation. Surety bonds are often required for durable medical equipment and patient's valuables. They may also be necessary to insure the following types of bonds: home health, residents' funds, performance and payment for construction contracts, notary, liquor, license, appeal and other court bonds, and pharmacy. Provider stop-loss coverage, on the other hand, prevents medical facilities from closing because of unforeseen and catastrophic loss. Medical facilities obtain stop-loss coverage to avoid having to pay losses over a certain amount per member annually. In some cases, stop-loss coverage is provided as part of the insurance provider's capitated agreement. It is also possible to purchase stop-loss coverage from commercial insurance carriers.

Due diligence before introducing new service models

Before introducing a new service model, healthcare facilities need to perform due diligence. The precise steps in this process will depend on the nature of the new process. If the process is new to this particular facility but is common elsewhere, the risk management department should discuss risks with the relevant employees at other facilities. If the service is entirely new, the risk management department may run simulations or conduct brainstorming sessions with stakeholders to identify possible areas of liability. The facility should concentrate on worst-case scenarios, as well as the possible magnifying effects of having several different errors occur in sequence. The facility should confer with its insurance provider to determine whether excess coverage should be purchased. Finally, the risk manager may want to contact the relevant professional association, as these bodies usually provide information as a general service to their members.

Legal and Regulatory

Negligence

Many of the adverse events that occur in healthcare facilities are the result of negligence rather than direct error. In law, an accusation of negligence must include four basic components: duty, breach of duty, cause of injury, and damages. First, the party accused of negligence must have had a clear duty to the wronged party. In healthcare, any provider who agrees to treat a patient has a demonstrable duty to that person. There must also be a breach of duty, meaning that the duty-bound party must have failed to meet the required standard of care or must have allowed hazardous conditions to exist. Third, an accusation of negligence requires that the plaintiff must have suffered a clear injury as a result of the breach of duty. Finally, this injury must be evidenced by specific damages, or demonstrable loss or adverse conditions suffered by the accusing party. Damages may include pain, medical expenses, or lost wages.

Liability issues for healthcare providers

General liability issues
Healthcare providers are subject to all of the liability issues faced by other businesses, as well as some others that are unique to the field. With respect to general liability, healthcare providers may be accused of negligence when the facility environment contains hazards, or when the patient suffers damages or loss caused by nonprofessional decisions and actions. A common example of a general negligence claim is when a patient falls on a wet floor that has not been properly marked. It is possible for a physician or other medical practitioner to be subject to a charge of negligence if the damages occur as a result of decisions, actions, or negligence that is not a part of the physician's professional practice. For this reason, charges of general liability do not need to be supported by expert testimony.

Medical professional liability issues
Healthcare providers must address the issue of medical professional liability. Medical professional liability differs from general liability in that it is the result of professional decisions made by medical practitioners during the delivery of service. A successful charge of medical negligence requires the four general elements of liability: duty, breach of duty, cause of injury, and damages. The duty which a medical practitioner owes to his or her patients is often known as the standard of care. It is common for an accusation of medical professional negligence to concentrate on establishing a definition for the standard of care and determining whether it has been met. Medical professional liability is sometimes referred to as malpractice liability.

Standard of care

In healthcare provision, standard of care is the required level of treatment that the practitioner owes to his or her patients. The precise definition of standard of care varies according to the circumstances, but a physician is generally expected to provide care commensurate with that provided by other practitioners in similar circumstances. In order to maintain a sufficient standard of care, then, the physician will need to stay abreast of advances in medical technique and equipment, and must be aware of his or her limitations as a practitioner. According to the "locality rule," physicians are judged relative to their peers in the same geographic area. However, in many states the basis for comparison is similar practitioners across the nation. If a physician presents him or herself as a specialist, however, he or she will be held to a higher standard. In the context of a negligence proceeding, the plaintiff will need to demonstrate the prevailing standard of care, and then prove that the physician failed to meet this standard.

Requirements for expert testimony

A healthcare professional must meet certain requirements to be qualified to deliver expert testimony in many states. To begin with, one must be licensed as a health professional in order to give testimony on medical subjects. An expert will also be expected to describe his or her education, training, and experience with respect to the subject of testimony. There are two common tests for a proposed witness. According to the Frye standard, which is used in many states, the expert opinion may be admitted as evidence if its underlying methodology is accepted by the professional community. According to the Daubert standard, which is used in many states and also at the federal level, the testimony may be admitted as evidence if it is supported by appropriate validation. Regardless of the standard used to support expert testimony, the expert will have to describe his or her level of certainty with respect to the testimony provided.

Negligence *per se* and privity

Healthcare institutions are required to confront the issue of negligence *per se* in situations where a statute clearly defines the standard of care. For instance, when a law is explicit about the appropriate conduct for a practitioner, it is unnecessary for the plaintiff to establish the standard of care as part of the trial. In other words, the plaintiff has a much easier time proving a duty and the breach of duty. Of course, the plaintiff must still demonstrate that the breach of duty was the cause of injury and that he or she suffered damages as a result. Another legal issue that relates to negligence cases is privity, or a mutual interest shared by the parties to a contract. A person or group who can demonstrate privity to the plaintiff in a negligence proceeding may be eligible for some compensation as well.

Duties of healthcare professionals regarding third parties

With respect to third parties, healthcare professionals cannot be charged with negligence in most states. That is, it has been established that the healthcare professional does not owe a duty to any third party. A third party, as for instance a relative or friend of the patient, cannot seek redress for damages suffered as a result of the treatment provided by the physician to the patient. There are some specific exceptions to this rule, as for instance when the patient's condition or behavior presents a clear risk to a third party. There are a few states in which doctors have a legal duty to third parties when the doctor is aware of a specific danger to the third party, or when the doctor has clear control over the patient. There are also some instances in which the doctor may be held liable for damages suffered by a third party who takes medication prescribed to a patient, especially if the doctor has failed to describe the risks of the medication to the patient at the time of prescription.

Contractual liability of doctors to patients

A doctor has a certain degree of contractual liability with respect to his or her patients. The amount of liability is determined in part by whether the contract is expressed or implied. An express contract is explicit, meaning that its terms are put into words and agreed upon by both parties. Also, an express contract includes consideration, meaning that each party must be receiving something of value. It is atypical for a physician to enter into an express contract with a patient, mostly because a medical practitioner cannot guarantee the success of a treatment protocol. An implied contract, on the other hand, exists whenever a medical practitioner agrees to treat a patient.

Informed consent

Healthcare institutions must frequently deal with issues related to informed consent. The relationship between the physician and the patient requires the consent of the patient. In legal terms, consent is typically defined as voluntary agreement to a proposition by another person. There are two categories of consent: general and informed. General consent is indicated by the presence of the patient in the examination room, but it only permits non-invasive procedures. In order to perform any invasive procedures, the practitioner needs to obtain informed consent, particularly when this procedure carries a material risk of harm. Informed consent requires that the patient be fully briefed on the nature of the procedure and its attendant risks, as well as any alternatives to the proposed treatment. Some people are not legally qualified to consent, as for instance minors.

Contractual negotiation and approval

Healthcare institutions are often called upon to handle issues related to contractual negotiation and approval. During the process of contract negotiation, the representatives of the healthcare institution must consider the requirements for each party: that is, what each party must do to fulfill the terms of the contract. The details of these requirements should be defined as narrowly as possible. For instance, the negotiators should agree about when and where the services will be provided. There should also be some standard for satisfactory performance. It is preferable for this metric to be clear, objective, and easy to obtain. In large healthcare facilities, it is especially important for the appropriate departments to be involved in the negotiation. For instance, purchasing contracts should be approved by the purchasing department as well as the financial department and general management.

Privilege and privacy issues

Peer review information
There are numerous privilege and privacy issues related to peer review information. This has been a tricky area for the courts to address because, while privacy must be respected, there is a clear value to having a peer review process whereby expert practitioners may evaluate each other's work. In several states, there are peer review protections that provide immunity to the members of these review boards and protection for documents created during the review process. Risk managers must become familiar with the rules in their jurisdiction. Moreover, people who provide information to peer review bodies are generally given protection from civil and criminal liability, so long as the information is within the scope of the report. People are also not protected if they knowingly provide false

information. Peer review protection extends to written documents as well as to conversations that take place within the peer review setting.

Patient confidentiality

There are numerous privilege and privacy issues related to patient confidentiality. Communication between a patient and doctor is considered confidential in every jurisdiction. If a physician unlawfully discloses confidential information, he or she may be subject to criminal or civil penalty. There are also federal laws prohibiting the wrongful disclosure of protected health information. Any person who obtains or discloses such information will be punished according to the severity of the offense. The penalty for a first offense is usually a $50,000 fine and imprisonment for one year. The punishment increases with each additional offense, or if the offense is committed under false pretenses. The punishment is most severe when the information is obtained or disclosed for malicious or commercial reasons.

Invoking attorney-client privilege

There are a few basic criteria for communications that have attorney-client privilege. To begin with, the party seeking protection must be an actual or prospective client. The communication must be between the actual or prospective client and an attorney acting as his or her legal counsel. The protected communication must have occurred without the presence of third parties, and must have been made in confidence. The communication must have been made to obtain a legal opinion. Furthermore, the party seeking attorney-client privilege must request it directly, and must not disclose the information to a third party, lest the privilege be waived. In the healthcare context, attorney-client privilege is most often invoked in the following circumstances: before potential litigation, while previous conduct is being investigated for possible legal relevance, when advice is being given about the structure of a new business, or during risk management and peer review.

Attorney-client privilege with written correspondence

The attorney-client privilege can be difficult to maintain with respect to memos and other written correspondence. To protect patients, the attorney is advised to head every relevant document with an indication of the attorney-client requirements. Documents should only be distributed to those parties who need to see them, and when not in use should be stored in a secure place. All document recipients should be indicated, i.e., there should be no blind copies. It should be noted that any information stored on hard drives, back-up systems, or disks is also subject to attorney-client privilege restrictions.

Joint Commission's efforts to prevent discrimination

The Joint Commission has established some specific recommendations that can help prevent discrimination. If a facility limits its selection criteria to certain characteristics, it should avoid problems with discrimination. For instance, medical staff should be required to adopt a set of bylaws that govern their conduct. Also, the medical staff should take deliberate steps to improve their performance through organization. The facility should have a clear and explicit policy for appointing, reappointing, and promoting staff members. The members of the staff should be authorized to monitor and evaluate the quality of patient care. The staff should also be required to participate in continuing education programs frequently. Finally, the staff should develop and implement a credentialing program for clinical privileges.

Impaired professional

The American Medical Association defines a professional as impaired when he or she cannot provide medical treatment with reasonable skill because of a mental or physical illness. This illness is not necessarily the result of drugs and/or alcohol: it may also be caused by aging, personal problems, or overwork. A healthcare facility has the responsibility to investigate and act appropriately whenever a practitioner is suspected to be impaired. The facility must remember at all times that the top priority is to provide quality medical care. Facilities are encouraged to draft their own protocols for handling impaired physicians. It is especially important for the facility to compile a report on the physician, and to file this report with the rehabilitation program. Rehabilitated professionals are allowed to return to practice, though there may be some rules of the Americans with Disabilities Act that pertain.

Ostensible or apparent agency

With respect to acute-care hospitals, ostensible or apparent agency may be applied if liability is incurred by an independent contractor. Ostensible agency exists if the patient seeks treatment from the institution as a whole, and the institution allows the contractor to provide the treatment on its behalf. Another condition of apparent agency is that the patient must have reason to assume that the contractor is an employee of the institution. If these criteria are met, the hospital can be held liable. This most often occurs when a patient is admitted to the emergency room, but there have also been situations in which pathologists, anesthesiologists, and radiologists have been negligent and the hospital has been held liable under the theory of ostensible agency.

Corporate negligence

The legal theory of corporate negligence asserts that hospitals have a duty to keep patients safe and well while they are under the institution's care. This duty cannot be delegated. It creates a meaningful distinction in the manner whereby a facility can be charged with negligence: when a patient is hurt by the negligence of a provider, the hospital is considered liable because it has failed to provide the appropriate standard of care, not because it is vicariously liable for the negligence itself. In order to justify a claim of corporate negligence against an acute-care hospital, the plaintiff must be able to prove that the hospital either knew or should have known about a procedural defect, and that the defect in question was a substantial reason for the patient's injury.

Legal issues specific to setting

<u>Continuing care retirement facilities and personal care homes</u>
There are a number of legal issues specific to continuing care retirement facilities and personal care homes. A continuing care retirement facility agrees to provide room, board, and medical care to residents for as long as they live. A continuing care retirement facility, often known as a CCRC, usually has several different departments that offer increasing levels of care. The liability issues to which such an institution is subject generally depend on whether independent and personal home care services or skilled nursing services are

provided. A personal care home, also known as an assisted living facility, is for patients who need a little less care. These institutions are typically administered by state agencies. In general, they are subject to much less regulation than nursing homes. As with CCRCs, the degree of liability is dependent on the level of care being provided. Both CCRCs and PCHs should be sure to provide as much care as necessary.

Nursing homes
There are a number of legal issues specific to nursing homes, which are licensed facilities that provide room, board, supervision, and personal assistance for patients who remain largely capable of caring for themselves. The care of nursing home residents is governed by the Omnibus Budget Reconciliation Act of 1987. This act outlines the requirements of care as well as the rights of residents. To receive Medicare and Medicaid payments, a nursing home must apply and be approved every nine to 15 months. Approval is based on performance with respect to four basic factors. The first of these is the quality of care furnished. This general heading includes physical activities, social participation, infection control, physical environment, sanitation, and nutrition. The other three factors are the adequacy of written plans of care, the accuracy of the resident's assessments, and compliance with the rights of residents.

Vicarious liability

The legal concept of vicarious liability has a somewhat unique application to healthcare institutions. All healthcare facilities may be held responsible for what their employees do or fail to do. The legal theory of vicarious liability is closely related to ostensible agency. Ostensible agency exists when a nursing home or other facility does not directly employ the practitioner at fault, but presents the practitioner to the patient as if the practitioner were an employee. For instance, a nursing home may enlist the services of a physician who, while technically not an employee of the nursing home, nevertheless represents the nursing home to the patient. In legal terms, the nursing home is said to "hold out" such a physician. If the courts determine that the facility has held out the practitioner, the courts may rule that the facility is vicariously liable for damages suffered by the plaintiff.

Corporate liability claims

The legal theory of corporate liability asserts that a healthcare facility has specific duties with respect to patients. If the facility fails to fulfill these duties, it may be held liable for any subsequent loss. The particular types of facilities that are subject to corporate liability claims have been debated in the courts over the past few years. There is a strong consensus that HMOs should be included in corporate liability claims, but there is not as yet a firm determination that nursing homes, hospitals, and long-term care facilities should always be included. In some situations, the courts may rule that the facility as a whole cannot be charged with liability, and that plaintiffs must instead bring charges against the individual practitioners involved.

Patient Self-Determination Act of 1990

The Patient Self-Determination Act of 1990 (PSDA) declares that a certain class of healthcare providers must give patients a standard set of information related to their future treatment. In particular, patients should be given the opportunity to make decisions about advance directives and end-of-life care. Each state has different rules about the extent to which patients may make decisions about their treatment should they become incapacitated or otherwise able to make decisions on their own behalf. According to the PSDA, each patient's medical record must include a copy of the relevant forms as well as an indication that the patient has been advised of his or her rights. The PSDA also asserts that care providers are not allowed to alter care in any way because of the patient's decisions in this respect. Finally, there are some staff education and training requirements outlined in the PSDA.

Advance directives in hospice care

An advance directive is a standard legal document in which a patient describes how he or she would like to be treated should he or she become unable to make decisions. The patient may either describe his or her preferred treatment protocol or may designate a person to act on his or her behalf. Advance directives are either durable powers of attorney or living wills. Durable powers of attorney are the designation of a surrogate for when the patient becomes unable to make decisions. A living will, on the other hand, is a declaration of the patient's preferences for the period immediately preceding his or her death. Each state has particular rules related to the drafting and maintenance of advance directives. The Patient Self-Determination Act of 1990 requires medical facilities to communicate the patient's rights with respect to advance directives.

Withholding or withdrawing life-sustaining treatment

The decision to withhold or withdraw life-sustaining treatment is affected by numerous legal issues. When there is no advance directive, the doctor must use his or her experience and knowledge of the case to make the best decision. This decision is especially fraught because continuing treatment against the wishes of the patient may be defined as invasive by the legal system, and the doctor could even be charged with battery. The American Medical Association (AMA) has attempted to aid the decision-making process by enumerating some basic factors that medical professionals should consider every time they must decide whether to withdraw treatment. The AMA asserts that professionals should consider the patient's averred attitude towards medical treatment and death, as well as the realistic potential for extending a worthwhile quality of life. Patients who are permanently unconscious may be ethically allowed to die, according to the AMA.

Duty to warn in mental and behavioral healthcare

The duty to warn in mental and behavioral healthcare is determined by a number of legal issues. Doctors are not allowed to share information acquired during treatment with third parties unless they have the consent of the patient. If a patient asserts his or her own mental incapacity, however, as for example in the context of a lawsuit, then the doctor has the right to disclose information. In addition, doctors have a duty to warn if they believe that a patient poses a threat to him or herself or to other people. There are some preconditions to this warning, however: the patient must have a defined target, and must have a clear and reasonable means of accomplishing his or her goal. It should be noted that the legalities surrounding the duty to warn vary from state to state, so risk managers must be familiar with the rules in their jurisdiction.

Responsibilities of hospital board

The hospital board has one major responsibility: to promote patient safety. This responsibility should take priority over any other duties of the board. So long as this responsibility is being met, however, the board may focus on its other responsibilities: maintaining the financial health of the institution and making improvements where necessary. The financial status of a healthcare institution is not totally distinct from its responsibility to promote patient safety, of course: if the institution has sufficient funds, it should be able to provide a high level of service. With respect to improvements within the institution, the board is responsible for ensuring that the facility offers the latest services, and that the patient outcomes are continuously improved.

Responsibilities of healthcare trustees

The members of the board of directors of a not-for-profit corporation are usually referred to as trustees. Trustees have two major duties: the duty of loyalty and the duty of care. For a trustee, being loyal means avoiding competition with the corporation, not disclosing confidential information about the corporation, and not taking any business away from the corporation. These are all part of the trustee's fiduciary obligation, or duty to act always in the best interests of the corporation. Finally, the duty of loyalty requires that trustees not enrich themselves at the expense of the corporation. The duty of care, meanwhile, binds trustees to act in good faith and in the best interests of the corporation at all times. Trustees are required to act in such a manner that a reasonable person would believe their actions to be good for the corporation.

Independent board members

The Panel on the Nonprofit Sector issued a report in 2005 entitled *Strengthening Transparency, Governance, and Accountability of Charitable Organizations*. This report made a number of recommendations that are applicable to the boards of healthcare institutions. One of these was that as many board members as possible should be independent. The Panel has a specific definition of independence for board members. A board member must not have been compensated by the organization within the past year, and must not have any aspect of his or her compensation determined by individuals who are affiliated with the organization. To be independent, a board member must not receive any material benefits from the organization and, moreover, must not be the husband, wife, brother, sister, parent, or child of any person who has received such benefits.

Disqualification from board service

The Panel report recommends specific protocols for disqualification from board service. To begin with, it recommends that any person who is prohibited by law from being on the boards of publicly traded companies or who has been convicted of a crime related to a breach of fiduciary duty should not be allowed to serve on the board of a charitable organization for five years. The report suggests that Congress should legislate this prohibition, but until this occurs, it is the responsibility of the organization and, more importantly, of the individual concerned to avoid such an appointment. It should be noted, however, that the Sarbanes-Oxley Act has given the Securities and Exchange Commission the authority to prevent specific people from serving on the boards of publicly traded companies.

Board compensation

With respect to board compensation, the Panel report indicated that the majority of board members for nonprofit healthcare organizations are not compensated. A charity or non-profit foundation does have every right to issue "reasonable compensation," however, to board members. Nevertheless, some people are disqualified from receiving compensation. For instance, any person who has been in a position to exercise substantial influence over the affairs of the organization in the past five years, or any member of such a person's family, is disqualified from serving on the board of a public charity. When it is necessary or appropriate to compensate board members, such compensation should be disclosed to the rest of the organization and the public as much as possible. In addition, the compensation should be based on comparisons with other organizations of a similar size and structure.

Educating the board of the healthcare organization

The risk management professional has some responsibility for educating the board of a healthcare organization. To begin with, the risk manager should ensure that the board of directors is familiar with the interrelationships among the quality improvement program, the medical staff credentialing program, and the risk management department. More generally, the board should understand the role and responsibilities of the risk manager, as well as the methods he or she uses to collect data and target risks. The board should know the highest areas of risk for the organization, as well as the source of most medical professional liability claims. The board should have access to the insurance policies held by the organization, as well as the claims history. Finally, and perhaps most importantly, the board should understand their role in preventing patient injury and minimizing liability.

Delivery of risk management information to the board of the healthcare organization

The protocol for delivering information about risk management to the board of the healthcare organization depends upon the size and structure of the organization. In most cases, the risk manager reports to the CEO, chief operating officer, or senior vice president. Sometimes, the risk manager will report to the vice president of medical affairs or the chief medical officer. In especially large organizations, the risk manager may report to a board committee, as for instance the professional affairs committee. In most of these arrangements, the board of directors receives its information from senior management rather than from the risk manager. One of the few cases in which a risk manager reports directly to the board of directors is if he or she is concerned that the managers are creating liability and/or putting patients at risk.

Communication with the board after Medicare and Medicaid fraud and abuse

After possible instances of Medicare and Medicaid fraud and abuse, the risk manager must communicate directly with the board. In the context of Medicare and Medicaid, fraud is defined as any intentional misrepresentations or knowingly false statements made in order to obtain a benefit. The most common types of Medicare and Medicaid fraud include accepting bribes, waiving copayments, making fraudulent diagnoses, billing for services that have not been provided, and forging records to justify payment. Besides Medicare and Medicaid fraud, any information related to the following should be communicated to the board as soon as possible: sentinel events and follow-up; payments, settlements, and

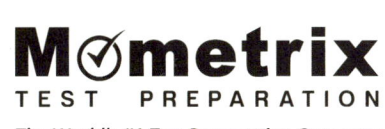

Dear Friend,

Thank you for ordering Mometrix products!

We take very seriously that you are entrusting your test preparation needs to us. We have meticulously prepared these materials to ensure we are offering you the most concise, relevant study aid possible. There are many resources available for your exam and we sincerely appreciate you choosing ours to help you attain the highest score within your ability to achieve.

You are about to experience an incredible transformation. Over the next few hours, days, weeks, or months of studying, you will transition from your current level of preparedness to an understanding of the exam content you never thought possible. You now hold in your hands the information you most need to know in order to succeed on your exam. Regardless of whether this is your first time to take the exam or your fifth time, our goal is to give you exactly what you need to maximize your score so you can go where you most want to go and be what you most want to be.

In addition to the products you have ordered from us, we have included a few bonuses that will help in your preparation. Be on the lookout for a special bonus website included in each product that offers additional tips and insights. In response to the test anxiety many people experience, we have also developed a free report to help you overcome this obstacle that you can access by visiting: www.mometrix.com/testanxiety.

From the many families here at Mometrix to yours, we sincerely thank you and wish you the best on your exam and every journey life has in store for you.

If you have any questions or suggestions as to how we can improve our products or service, please contact us at 800-673-8175 or support@mometrix.com.

Sincerely,

Jay Willis
Vice President of Sales
Mometrix Test Preparation

P.S. - We would greatly appreciate you recommending our products to your friends and colleagues!

judgments; quality trends; inquiries related to the death of a patient; and any lawsuits filed, the nature of claims, and the steps being taken to address concerns about quality.

Content and format of reports to the board of the healthcare organization

The reports submitted by a risk manager to the board of the healthcare organization must have standard content and format. The risk manager wants to provide all of the important information without overwhelming the board with data. Every report should contain a concise summary, in plain language, of the current status. Many institutions ask the risk manager to include what is known as a consent agenda, which is a list of routine requests and notifications about which the board should be informed, but which are not likely to require debate. The presence of a consent agenda expedites the board's handling of the risk management matters. It is also a good idea for the reports to include a standard list of indicators so that the members of the board can track the performance of the risk management department over time. Some of the indicators that are typically found in reports to the board are number of claims, cost of claims, and the results of insurance audits. It is also very important for a risk manager to present his or her findings at least in part in a graphic format, as non-experts will find this presentation more accessible.

Development of a medical staff development plan

The medical staff development plan is an explanation of the specific policies that the organization will use to help staff members fulfill the overall mission of the institution. The first step is for the board of directors to adopt a basic resolution to create the development plan, and to outline a basic statement of community service principles. The physicians placed in charge of developing the medical staff development plan should not have any economic conflicts of interest. The next step is for the physicians who have been conducting the research to communicate their findings with the remaining members of the institution. This gives the rest of the community a chance to provide feedback. Then, the staff development plan team will collect more information about the needs of the community. This might include general demographic data as well as more specific medical information, like number of emergency room visits and average wait for patients. The staff development plan team should also take a look at the financial relationships of the management and employees of the institution with an eye towards discovering conflicts of interest and opportunities for synergy. Finally, the team will make its recommendations and, after some debate, a plan will be drafted and adopted by the board.

Reporting requirements for workplace violence

The reporting requirements related to violence in the workplace vary by state. However, some states have yet to pass legislation that directly addresses this issue. Depending on the intended strategy for handling this problem, the laws that have been passed can generally be divided into two categories. First, there are laws that seek to prevent violence in the workplace before it occurs. Some of these laws address all workplaces, while others, as for instance the Illinois Health Care Workplace Violence Prevention Act, are specific to the field of healthcare. The Illinois law requires employers to create a specific plan, and to review it at least every three years. Other laws, like the California Workplace Violence Safety Act, take a retrospective approach to workplace violence: that is, they give authority to employers to punish and even issue restraining orders against perpetrators. Despite the differences in approach between these laws, they all impose specific reporting requirements on employers. Indeed, in some cases there are penalties for employers who fail to report incidents of violence in the workplace.

Investigation and resolution of patient complaints

Each state has specific requirements for the investigation and resolution of patient complaints. In a typical arrangement, patient complaints are immediately acknowledged in writing, at which point the state health department will conduct an initial investigation. If there is reason to believe that a violation has occurred, the department will conduct an unannounced investigation at the healthcare facility. At this time, the health department may require the patient to submit more information, whether in writing or in a formal interview. Also, the healthcare facility will be invited to submit an account of the incident. In some cases, the investigation will be combined with the already scheduled inspection of the healthcare facility. In any case, once the complaint has been fully investigated, both the complainant and the healthcare facility will receive a ruling on the subject, including any relevant punishments for the institution.

Federal sentencing guidelines

The federal sentencing guidelines for healthcare organizations are maintained by the United States Sentencing Commission. These guidelines apply to both non-profit and for-profit organizations. According to the guidelines, the authority that governs the organization should be familiar with the relevant compliance and ethics program, and should exercise any necessary influence over this program. In most cases, this authority is the board of directors or some other executive body. Organizations are charged with conducting any training necessary to ensure that employees understand their responsibilities. The intention of the federal sentencing guidelines is to standardize the punishments for common offenses, whether committed by individuals or corporations.

Sarbanes-Oxley Act of 2002

The Sarbanes-Oxley Act of 2002 was the legislative response to the rash of business scandals in the early years of the 21st century. The act is not directly applicable to nonprofit hospitals and healthcare facilities, but many medical organizations have elected to comply with the act as a simple matter of good practice. One of the requirements of the Sarbanes-Oxley Act is that senior executives must personally vouch for financial statements. Also, directors and officers are forbidden from misleading the general public or a certified accountant in any way. Another product of the Sarbanes-Oxley Act was the Accounting Oversight Board, which is responsible for monitoring corporate auditors. Although this body does not exercise any influence over healthcare organizations as such, it remains important for these organizations to avoid conflicts of interest with monitoring bodies. Moreover, the Sarbanes-Oxley Act requires corporations to announce any changes in financial condition or operations, and healthcare organizations would be wise to follow these requirements as well.

Volunteer Protection Act of 1997

The Volunteer Protection Act of 1997 was originally intended to protect volunteers at nonprofit organizations, but it is broad enough to apply to the trustees of healthcare organizations. According to the act, the trustees of a healthcare organization are protected from excessive liability and punitive action stemming from actions committed during the course of their volunteer work. Specifically, trustees cannot be held liable for actions that are a part of their work as a volunteer. The only exceptions are for actions that are caused by "willful or criminal misconduct, gross negligence, reckless misconduct, or a conscious, flagrant indifference to the rights or safety of the individual harmed by the volunteer." The claimant is responsible for proving that the volunteer was the proximate cause of the harm.

Administrative Procedure Act

The Administrative Procedure Act is the blueprint for federal rule making and enforcement. When an agency wants to create a new rule, it must first publish a notice in the *Federal Register*. Then there is an interval of at least 30 days in which the general public is allowed to comment and to request more information about the proposed rule. Once the rule has been finalized, it is again published in the *Federal Register*, along with a summary of the changes that have been made since the original rule proposal. Once a rule has gone into effect, the responsibility for enforcing it lies with the issuing agency. Agencies are allowed to use permit approvals, fines, and penalties to support the rules. Agencies are allowed to call hearings to adjudicate complications of the rules, and the results of these hearings may be appealed by the participants.

Administrative enforcement

In healthcare, the two primary organizations with responsibility for enforcing safety and environmental laws are the Occupational Safety and Health Administration (OSHA) and the Environmental Protection Agency (EPA). Each of these organizations can levy significant fines and penalties against violators of their regulations. OSHA prefers for institutions to obey the law of their own accord, so it has established a voluntary protection program under which the institution can pass a strict evaluation and subsequently be exempt from regular inspections. Another option for cooperative businesses is the strategic partnership program, in which OSHA acts as a facilitator and expert resource for an institution or an industry looking to resolve a particular safety issue. For all other institutions, however, regular inspections are necessary. These inspections may be scheduled, as in the case of serious violations or complaints, or unscheduled. An inspection may be limited to certain high hazard areas or operations of the institution, or it may be comprehensive.

OSHA inspection

When an OSHA inspector arrives at an institution, the employer does have the right to demand an inspection warrant unless there is a known hazard that is placing employees at risk of harm. An OSHA inspector is allowed to subpoena any necessary records, documents, or testimony. For instance, the inspector may want to gather some information related to exposure records, illness/injury, or the lockout-tagout program. The inspection usually begins with a brief conference among the inspector, employer, and employees. Then, the inspector will roam around the facility and collect samples, measurements, and photographs. OSHA inspectors also have the authority to interview employees in private, either on or off the premises. After the inspection, the inspector may issue a citation, which may include requirements that have to be fulfilled by the employer within a certain interval.

Major substances and practices regulated by OSHA

The Occupational Safety and Health Administration (OSHA) requires employers to maintain a safe working environment for their employees. To this end, the organization has a list of substances and practices that are subject to regulation. The major substances and practices regulated by OSHA are acetone; ethyl, isopropyl, and methyl alcohol; asbestos; benzene; bloodborne pathogens; cadmium; confined space entry; ethylene oxide; formaldehyde; hazard communications; hazardous waste operations and emergency response; hydrogen peroxide; laboratory standards; lead; lockout-tagout rule; mercury; methyl methacrylate; noise; personal protective equipment; toluene; tuberculosis exposure; and xylene. These are all recognized hazards that could pose a danger to employees. OSHA also has regulations related to walking surfaces, work areas, ladders, and welding.

Major health issues regulated by the EPA

Some major health issues are regulated by the Environmental Protection Agency (EPA), especially those related to outdoor materials and activities. Whereas the Occupational Safety and Health Administration has individual health as its primary focus, the EPA is more interested in protecting larger groups through the regulation of pollution. There are a number of specific statutes that elaborate the powers of the EPA. For instance, the Comprehensive Environmental Response, Compensation, and Liability Act (also known as the Superfund) forces landowners to pay for the cleanup costs on contaminated lands. The EPA is very aggressive about pursuing compensation on Superfund sites. The Resource Conservation and Recovery Act, meanwhile, allows the EPA to manage the disposal of solid and hazardous waste, including the use of underground storage tanks. The Clean Air Act gives the EPA the authority to regulate the incineration of medical waste and to establish the national ambient air quality standards. The Toxic Substances Control Act gives the EPA the authority to regulate the toxic chemicals used in the industry.

Major health issues not specifically regulated by OSHA

There are some major health issues that are not specifically regulated by the Occupational Safety and Health Administration (OSHA). However, this does not mean that there are no other risks to healthcare workers besides those regulated by the government. For instance, the following issues are not addressed by OSHA regulations: compressed gases, ergonomics and musculoskeletal disorders, extremely low-frequency electric and magnetic fields, flammable liquids, glutaraldehyde, hazardous drugs, indoor air quality, lasers, laser or electrocautery plume, latex sensitivity, mold and fungus, radiation, video display terminals, waste anesthetic gases, and workplace violence. There are health risks associated with all of these issues, and risk managers should be very familiar with them. In some instances, substances and processes that are not addressed by OSHA regulations are monitored by the Environmental Protective Agency.

Development of new metrics

Risk managers should always be alert for opportunities to improve their self-assessment by creating better metrics. To be effective, however, a metric must have the following characteristics: sensitivity, quantifiability, uniqueness, feasibility, validity, reliability, baseline, and multidimensionality. Sensitivity is the extent to which the measured item responds to risk management activities. The meaningfulness of the metric is the degree to which it relates to a key aspect of the program. The uniqueness of the metric is the extent to which it measures a specific and isolated component of the program. The realm of control is the extent to which the factor can be affected by the conscious actions of the risk management department. Feasibility is the ease with which the data can be collected. Validity is the extent to which the metric measures what it was intended to measure. Reliability is the extent to which the results of the measurement can be replicated by different users at different times. A baseline is a comparison measurement against which the new data can be compared. Finally, multidimensionality is the extent to which the metric provides information about several different aspects of the process.

Major licensure, accreditation, and certification activities

Most healthcare facilities are required by law to obtain organizational licensure. In addition, healthcare professionals are required to get individual licensure, and some employees will require specific licensure because of their job responsibilities. Whereas licensure activities are often mandatory, accreditation and certification activities are more likely to be optional. Another difference is that licensure activities are usually administered by a governmental body, while accreditation and certification activities are run by industry-wide or other private organizations. Risk managers are typically responsible for overseeing the licensure, accreditation, and certification activities of their employer. This entails staying abreast of any deadlines and mandatory standards.

Vendor liability programs

Medical facilities must implement vendor liability programs to handle any problems that arise because of errors made by the providers of medical equipment or supplies. A large part of a vendor liability program is the acquisition of specific vendor liability insurance coverage, usually acquired as an addition to the general liability policy. This insurance covers the medical facility against the possibility of becoming liable for injury or illness caused by errors made by a vendor. Some insurance carriers will only offer limited coverage as part of a vendor liability policy, in part because the medical facility will often escape liability for problems arising from the actions of a third party. The vendor liability program should also include a summary of the licensures required by the vendors of specialized or high-risk products. For instance, pharmaceutical manufacturers and vendors are required to hold specific licenses and permits for handling and distributing their products. The risk manager should verify these licenses and permits frequently, and according to a regular schedule.

Centers for Medicare and Medicaid Services

Every year, the Centers for Medicare and Medicaid Services (CMS) spend over $500 million to administer the Medicare, Medicaid, and State Children's Health Insurance Programs. For many healthcare facilities, CMS payments amount to over half of total income. The CMS has established the following standing committees to address specific issues in healthcare: Practicing Physicians Advisory Council, Advisory Panel on Medicare Education, Medicare Coverage Advisory Committee, Advisory Panel on Ambulatory Payment Classification Groups, Competitive Pricing Advisory Committee, Emergency Medical Treatment and Labor Act Technical Advisory Group, Advisory Board on the Demonstration of a Bundled Case-Mix Adjusted Payment System for End-stage Renal Disease Services, Medicaid Commission, and the State Pharmaceutical Assistance Transition Committee. The CMS also works with quality improvement organizations and administers its own set of compliance programs.

Roles in surveying healthcare organizations

Department of Health and Human Services
The Department of Health and Human Services (HHS) is the primary instrument of the United States government for providing health services. In particular, the HHS focuses on distributing health services to the disadvantaged. The HHS collaborates on hundreds of projects with state and local governments, and has 11 distinct operating divisions: Administration for Children and Families, Administration on Aging, Agency for Healthcare Research and Quality, Agency for Toxic Substances and Disease Registry, Centers for Disease Control and Prevention, Centers for Medicare and Medicaid Services, Food and Drug Administration, Health Resources and Services Administration, Indian Health Service, National Institutes of Health, and Substance Abuse and Mental Health Services Administration. For most people, the face of the HHS is the Centers for Medicare and Medicaid Services, which deliver health insurance to more than 80 million Americans.

State health department
Each state has a health department that is responsible for monitoring the care providers that operate within its borders. These agencies range from very aggressive to laissez-faire, depending upon the regulatory culture in the state. In most states, however, there is a specific set of activities for which the state health department is responsible. The state health department typically performs regular inspections, emergency management, and standard-setting in cooperation with private accrediting bodies. The extent to which the state health department collaborates with other organizations on its inspection program varies. In some cases, the state collaborates with the Joint Commission and the state medical association. Also, it is common for states to focus their inspections on the most important activities, as for instance the review of credentials.

Joint Commission
The Joint Commission on Accreditation for Healthcare Organizations, commonly known simply as the Joint Commission, was formed in 1951 by the American College of Surgeons, Canadian Medical Association, American Medical Association, American Hospital Association, and American College of Physicians. The Joint Commission is a private nonprofit primarily focused on ameliorating organized healthcare in the United States and Canada. Specifically, the Joint Commission accreditation programs are the industry gold standard. After the applying healthcare provider completes a survey, the Joint Commission will issue accreditation, provisional accreditation, a conditional accreditation, preliminary denial of accreditation, or denial of accreditation. A preliminary denial of accreditation may be appealed. According to the Joint Commission, accreditation results in improved patient care; enhanced safety and quality improvement efforts; a demonstration of the organization's commitment to safety and quality; a consultative and educational experience; strengthened recruitment and retention efforts; substitution for federal certification surveys for Medicare and Medicaid; secured managed care contracts; facilitation of the organization's business strategies; competitive advantage; enhanced image to the public, purchasers, and payers; fulfilment of licensure requirements in many states; recognition by insurers and other third parties; and strengthened community confidence.

AOA and NCQA

The American Osteopathic Association (AOA) issues accreditation to healthcare facilities in the United States. The AOA is authorized by the Centers for Medicare and Medicaid Services to monitor hospitals according to the Conditions of Participation in Medicare. This monitoring is mainly conducted by survey, which is conducted on location at the healthcare facility. The AOA has developed specific standards to be used in facilities for physical rehabilitation, substance abuse, mental health, and ambulatory care and surgery. The National Committee for Quality Assurance (NCQA), meanwhile, is responsible for monitoring managed care plans. Specifically, the NCQA provides information to consumers of managed healthcare. While being surveyed by the NCQA, managed care plans are required to provide data related to access and service to the plan; qualified providers in the plan; preventive health measures; effective treatments, drugs, and devices; and the management of chronic illness.

HEDIS and the ISO 9001:2000

The National Committee for Quality Assurance developed the Health Plan Employer Data and Information Set (HEDIS) to facilitate the comparison of health plans. This system organizes healthcare providers according to 50 basic measures of performance. For instance, the HEDIS system generates statistics about member satisfaction, immunization rates, and the management of key health determinants (as for instance cholesterol). The ISO 9001:2000, meanwhile, is the set of standards established by the International Organization for Standardization (ISO). The American National Standards Institute (ANSI) represents the United States at the ISO. The general goal of ISO standards is to increase the collection of data and the documentation of processes. According to the ISO, healthcare facilities that adopt the standards are better able to comply with customer requirements for ISO 9001:2000, compete in global and domestic markets, improve the existing quality management system, minimize repetitive auditing by accrediting organizations, and improve subcontractor and vendor performance. Moreover, the benefits to participating organizations include enhanced understanding of quality management throughout the organization, a mechanism to improve documentation of process and procedures, a tool to strengthen and improve supplier and customer confidence, cost savings and improved profitability, improved organizational awareness of quality, and strengthened continuous performance improvement.

College of American Pathologists and Clinical Laboratories Quality Standards program

The College of American Pathologists is an international professional organization for physicians and laboratories. It is the acknowledged leader in programs to improve laboratory quality. The Clinical Laboratories Quality Standards program is the arm of the Centers for Medicare and Medicaid Services that monitors any laboratory research performed on humans. Laboratories that only perform simple procedures may obtain a waiver from specific Clinical Laboratory Improved Amendments (CLIA) requirements. Only the following laboratory procedures are exempt from specific CLIA standards: dipstick or tablet urinalysis, fecal occult blood, ovulation test using visual color comparison, urine pregnancy test using visual color comparison, erythrocyte sedimentation rate, hemoglobin by copper sulfate method, spine micro hematocrit, blood glucose using certain devices cleared by the FDA specifically for home use, and whole blood hemoglobin assays. Facilities that obtain a waiver will not be inspected very often.

CARF

The Commission on Accreditation of Rehabilitation Facilities (CARF) is a major accreditation organization for medical rehabilitation, community services, employment, adult day services, and behavioral health. The mission of this organization is to create and maintain quality standards in these areas. According to CARF, the preeminent goals of covered facilities should be the continuous improvement of organizational management and service delivery; diversity and cultural competency in all CARF activities and associations; recognizing organizations that are accredited through a consultative peer review process; conducting accreditation research; and providing consultation, education, training, and publications that promote accreditation. The Continuing Care Accreditation Commission, which is the accrediting component of the Commission on Accreditation of Rehabilitation Facilities, assesses facilities on the basic of six criteria: assessing the environment; strategy development; person-served focus; implementing the plan, processes, and programs for the person served; reviewing results; and evaluating the results and progress of a strategy.

AAAASF

The American Association for Accreditation of Ambulatory Surgery Facilities (AAAASF) is a voluntary program for the advancement of surgery facilities in the United States. Although this organization originally arose to monitor plastic surgery facilities, its purview now includes any office-based surgery facilities. The AAAASF defines the major areas of office-based ambulatory surgery practice as follows: general environment; operating room environment, policy, and procedures; recovery room environment, policy, and procedures; general safety in the facility; blood and medications; medical records; quality assessment and improvement; personnel; and governance. One of the unique features of the AAAASF is that it employs working surgeons, nurses, and anesthesiologists as its surveyors.

URAC

The Utilization Review Accreditation Commission (URAC), sometimes known as the American Accreditation HealthCare Commission, is a collective that is devoted to creating and maintaining standards for the managed care industry. URAC receives contributions from regulators, healthcare providers, employers, and consumers. There are 22 certification and accreditation programs offered for managed healthcare organizations: case management, claims processing, consumer education and support, core accreditation, credentials support certification, credentials verification organization (CVO), disease management, drug therapy management, health call center, health content and personal health management providers accreditation, health network, health plan, health provider credentialing, health utilization management, health web site, HIPAA privacy, HIPAA security, independent review organization, Medicare advantage deeming program, primary benefit management, vendor certification, and workers compensation utilization management.

CHAP

The Community Health Accreditation Program (CHAP) is the primary accrediting body for the home care industry. According to CHAP, home care organizations must meet the following four general requirements: the structure and function of the organization should consistently support its consumer-oriented philosophy and purpose; the organization should consistently provide high-quality services and products; the organization should have sufficient human, financial, and physical resources appropriately organized to accomplish the intended purpose; and the organization should be situated to be viable over the long term. CHAP has established specific standards for the following facilities: adult day care services, community nursing centers, community rehabilitation centers, home care aide services, home dialysis services, home health services, home infusion therapy, home medical equipment, hospice care, pharmacy services, private duty nursing, public health services, and supplemental staffing.

NCCHC and CODA

The National Commission on Correctional Health Care (NCCHC) is responsible for maintaining standards for the provision of healthcare in correctional facilities. Anyone who works in a correctional facility is eligible to receive accreditation from the NCCHC. A recent focus of the NCCHC has been the rash of opiate abuse in correctional facilities. The NCCHC is open to many different types of professionals, including nurses, physicians, mental health workers, dentists, attorneys, health information technicians, and administrators. Programs that are accredited by the NCCHC are able to apply for accreditation by the Substance Abuse and Mental Health Services Administration. The Commission on Dental Accreditation (CODA), which is run by the American Dental Association, is responsible for creating and maintaining professional standards in dentistry and dental education. CODA has established professional standards in these areas: dental public health, endodontics, general dentistry, general practice residency, oral and maxillofacial pathology, oral and maxillofacial radiology, oral and maxillofacial surgery, orthodontics and dentofacial orthopedics, pediatric dentistry, periodontics, and prosthodontics.

US FDA

The United States Food and Drug Administration (FDA) is a consumer protection agency charged with monitoring the manufacture, import, transport, storage, and sale of billions of dollars of products every year. The FDA is a component of the public health service, which itself is a part of the Department of Health and Human Services. In general, the FDA monitors the following product categories: food, cosmetics, medicines, medical devices, blood supply, radiation emitting products, animal feed, and animal drugs. It does so through inspections and legal sanctions. If a product is considered unsafe and presents an immediate threat to the general public, then the FDA has the authority to initiate a recall. The FDA also has the authority to impose criminal penalties against distributors and manufacturers who violate the regulations.

EEOC

The United States Equal Employment Opportunity Commission (EEOC) was created by Title VII of the Civil Rights Act of 1964. The general mission of the EEOC is the prevention of discrimination through education and outreach, voluntary resolution of disputes when possible, and strong and fair enforcement when resolution fails. These goals are outlined in the National Enforcement Plan, which was issued by the EEOC in 1996. The EEOC is responsible for enforcing Title VII of the Civil Rights Act of 1964, the Equal Pay Act of 1963, the Age Discrimination in Employment Act of 1967, Title I of the Americans with Disabilities Act of 1990, the Civil Rights Act of 1991, and Section 501 of the Rehabilitation Act of 1973. In addition, the EEOC runs technical assistance programs and provides support to state and municipal fair employment practices agencies.

ISO 9001:2000 Quality Systems Standard

The ISO 9001:2000 Quality Systems Standard is a series of performance requirements for the organizations that make up the healthcare delivery system. The major requirements of the ISO 9001 Standards are as follows: quality management systems; documentation requirements; quality manuals; control of documents and records; management responsibility; management commitment; customer focus; quality policy; planning; quality objectives; responsibility, authority, and communication; internal communication; resource management; provision of resources; human resources; competence, awareness, and training; infrastructure; work environment; planning of product realization; customer related processes; determination of requirements related to the product; customer communication; design and development planning, inputs, outputs, review, verification, and validation; control of design and development changes; purchasing; production and service provision; identification and traceability; customer property; preservation of product; and the control of monitoring and measuring devices.

ISO registration

There are four phases in the ISO registration. In Phase I, Organizing for Registration, the facility will obtain management commitment, establish a steering committee, begin internal quality auditing, and select a registrar. In Phase II, Preparing for Registration, the facility must document existing processes with procedures and work instructions, identify areas that need improvement, adopt improved procedures and work instructions, prepare the quality manual, apply to the registrar for an assessment, consider a pre-assessment, conduct a dress rehearsal audit, submit the revised manual to the registrar, modify and finalize quality practices, and train personnel. During Phase III, Experiencing the ISO Registration Audit, the facility must arrange for the registrar to conduct the assessment and identify findings (discrepancies), respond to findings, submit to the registrar for review the proposed corrective actions, and receive the registration certificate. Finally, in Phase IV, Continuing ISO Registration through Surveillance Audits, the facility must maintain quality practice to ensure continuing compliance, notify the registrar of major changes in practice, arrange for the registrar to conduct semiannual surveillance audits, and continue to improve.

Emergency Medical Treatment and Labor Act

The Emergency Medical Treatment and Labor Act of 1986, also called the "antidumping law" or COBRA, prevents medical facilities from denying treatment to patients who cannot pay. Previously, it had been standard practice in many states to transfer indigent patients from emergency rooms to public hospitals. In order to receive Medicare subsidies, a hospital must provide any necessary diagnostic and therapeutic services to identify emergency medical conditions. Moreover, hospitals are required to clinically stabilize any medical condition that may be an immediate threat to the health of the patient and, if the required resources are not available, the hospital is required to transfer the patient to another facility. Patients should be aware of their rights under the Emergency Medical Treatment and Labor Act and, indeed, hospitals are required to post notice of these rights in a prominent location. It should be noted that the obligation of the hospital to provide screening and stabilizing services does not obviate the debt of the patient, i.e., the medical facility is still owed payment for whatever service it provides.

Implications for risk management
The Emergency Medical Treatment and Labor Act has specific implications for risk management. This act was part of the Consolidated Omnibus Budget Reconciliation Act of 1986. The intention of the act was to prevent emergency departments from refusing service

to indigent patients. According to the act, any person who comes to a hospital in need of evaluation or treatment must be provided with any diagnostic or therapeutic services that are required to identify the presence of an emergency medical condition, to stabilize any condition that is an immediate threat to the patient, and to transfer the patient to a fully equipped hospital if more care is necessary. It should be noted that while the law does forbid healthcare facilities from denying treatment to those who cannot pay, it does not prevent them from billing these patients. In accordance with this law, hospitals must maintain a central log of every person who arrives at the facility for evaluation or treatment. Emergency departments must also maintain a record of the healthcare professionals who are available to treat those patients who fall under the provisions of this act.

Medicare Modernization Act

The Medicare Modernization Act of 2003 outlines a policy for compensating hospitals that provide services under the Emergency Medical Treatment and Labor Act (EMTALA). A large fund has been set aside by the federal government for this reason. However, before receiving any of these funds, the healthcare facility needs to demonstrate that it has attempted to receive payment from the patient, insurance providers, and any government alternative payment plans. One of the problems for risk managers with respect to this act is to identify those patients who are qualified to receive free care without discriminating. The risk manager should be sure that the screening process does not discourage the prospective patient from seeking treatment. If a risk manager determines that a significant enough percentage of patients are eligible for EMTALA care, then he or she may wish to apply for funds under the Medicare Modernization Act of 2003.

Health Care Quality Improvement Act

The Health Care Quality Improvement Act of 1986 was part of an effort to improve the quality of care and reduce the number of medical malpractice suits. One of the major components of the legislation was the creation of a peer review system for dentists, physicians, and other healthcare practitioners. To promote this system, the federal government agreed to grant broad legal immunity to professionals to contribute to it. For risk managers, it is essential to learn how the implementation and cultivation of a peer review system can limit the number and severity of claims made against the organization. For instance, the practitioners may gain some degree of confidentiality, or may be granted immunity from discovery related to civil litigation. On the other hand, a risk management department can forfeit these protections by failing to abide by the appropriate regulations related to the retention and release of patient information.

National Practitioner Data Bank

The National Practitioner Data Bank is another product of the Health Care Quality Improvement Act. This is a collection of all the complaints registered against physicians and other healthcare practitioners. Whenever a practitioner is found guilty of professional negligence or settles a lawsuit of this type, several sources of information about the incident are compiled into a database entry. In addition, hospitals are required to notify their state board whenever a physician voluntarily relinquishes his or her medical staff privileges as a response to the threat of disciplinary action, or whenever the hospital limits a practitioner's staff membership or clinical privileges for a period of at least 30 days. Whenever a hospital processes an application for medical staff membership, it is required to submit a query to the National Practitioner Data Bank. Moreover, facilities must submit such queries every two years subsequent to the granting of membership privileges. Practitioners may query the National Practitioner Data Bank about themselves at any time, but the database will not provide any information to medical malpractice insurers, defense attorneys, or members of the general public.

HIPDB

The Healthcare Integrity and Protection Data Bank (HIPDB) is one of the products of the Health Insurance Portability and Accountability Act of 1996. To avoid confusion with the National Practitioner Data Bank, the HIPDB has been linked to that database via the Integrated Querying and Reporting System. For risk managers, the most important factors related to the HIPDB are compliance with the investigation and reporting requirements. The penalties for failure to comply with the confidentiality provisions of the law can be very severe. At the same time, there is wide speculation that hospitals do not report to the HIPDB as often as they should. There is growing support for even harsher penalties for delinquent organizations.

Patient Self-Determination Act of 1990

The Patient Self-Determination Act of 1990, a component of the Omnibus Budget Reconciliation Act, established a new set of standards for end-of-life decisions. Specifically, it asserted that competent patients have the right to make legally enforceable and binding decisions about how their healthcare should be handled if they become incapacitated. This act applies to hospitals, home healthcare services, health maintenance organizations, hospice programs, and skilled nursing facilities; it does not apply to private physicians' offices or freestanding outpatient clinics. An advance directive is defined as a lawful written instruction, as for instance a living will or designation of power of attorney. One of the intentions of the law was to encourage more patients to make these decisions earlier. Risk managers should take every reasonable step to encourage patients to make advance directives, though it is illegal to deny service or make care inaccessible to those patients who decline to do so.

Medicare treatment of patients' rights

Beginning in 1999, Medicare began enforcing a set of six standards related to patients' rights. These standards apply to acute-care hospitals, psychiatric hospitals, psychiatric treatment units, and skilled nursing facilities. To begin with, hospitals are required to notify every patient (or patient's representative) before care is initiated or discontinued. At the very least, the hospital should have a specific protocol for where, when, and how patients are to be provided with this information. Also, every hospital should have a policy for handling patient complaints related to the failure to provide notification. When a patient registers such a grievance, he or she should be given the name of a contact person at the hospital, as well as a description of the steps taken during the investigation of the complaint, the results of this investigation, and the date on which the investigation was performed. However, the Medicare guidelines are somewhat vague on this issue, so it is the responsibility of the risk manager to ensure that the facility is in compliance.

Medicare standards related to patients' rights

<u>Exercise of rights, privacy, safety, and confidentiality</u>
According to Medicare, medical facilities are required to advise patients that they have the right to participate in the creation of their treatment plans. In addition, patients should be advised that they have the right to make informed decisions related to their course of treatment. Medicare establishes that patients have the right to be informed continually about their health status. Finally, the standards assert that patients have the right to create their own advance directives and to have these followed by the medical staff. The Medicare standards also assert that patients have the right to personal privacy, as well as to receive care in a safe environment where they will not be troubled by harassment, abuse, or harm. The Medicare standards also reassert the confidentiality requirements issued by HIPAA and the respective states. Patient information is protected, and must be retained by the healthcare facility for a specified interval.

<u>Restraints in acute medical and surgical care, seclusion, and restraint</u>
Medicare has established a definition for restraint and has outlined when it can be used in acute medical and surgical care. These rules must be explicitly taught to staff, and this training must be refreshed regularly. Moreover, hospitals need to maintain accurate records of employee attendance at this training, in case they are later called upon to prove that employees have received the training. The Medicare patients' rights standards also cover specifically the use of seclusion and restraint for behavior management in psychiatric care settings. According to the Medicare guidelines, hospitals need to enlist the services of a licensed independent practitioner to determine whether the patient requires restraint or seclusion. The licensed independent practitioner should be given the opportunity to evaluate the patient within one hour of the beginning of seclusion or restraint.

Medicare Conditions of Participation with respect to infection control and nursing services

The Medicare Condition of Participation related to infection control asserts that every facility must designate an infection control officer and implement policies that are targeted at controlling infection and communicable disease. Furthermore, facilities are required to maintain a log of such conditions, and the chief executive officer, medical staff, and director of nursing services are responsible for ensuring that the infection control program is implemented and monitored. The Medicare Condition of Participation related to nursing services, meanwhile, covers a broad range of issues on this topic. For instance, it has recommendations related to staffing, the development of nursing care plans, medication administration, adverse drug reactions, reporting blood transfusion reactions, and staff competency assessment.

Safe Medical Devices Act of 1990

The Safe Medical Devices Act of 1990 gives the Food and Drug Administration (FDA) the authority to collect information about medical device safety. In particular, the FDA is responsible for collecting information about adverse incidents related to medical devices. There are specific reporting requirements for the manufacturers of all medical devices. A detailed account of these recommendations is published by the Office of Surveillance and Biometrics, a part of the FDA's Center for Devices and Radiological Health. The Safe Medical Devices Act applies to nursing homes, home healthcare agencies, rescue squads, hospitals, ambulatory surgical facilities, ambulance providers, rehabilitation facilities, psychiatric facilities, and any outpatient diagnostic and treatment facilities that are not physicians' offices. The act does not apply to freestanding care units, dental offices, physicians, optometrists, nurse practitioners, chiropractors, and employee health clinics.

Reporting, medical device tracking, and reusable single-use devices
The Safe Medical Devices Act of 1990 requires the users of medical devices to notify the manufacturer within 10 days of learning about a serious patient injury or death related to the use of the device. Users are asked to file the MedWatch form provided by the Food and Drug Administration (FDA). If a patient's death is related to the use of the medical device, the FDA must be notified as well. Also, medical facilities must provide the FDA with a summary list of all the medical device reports it has made in the past year. Medical facilities are required to maintain these records for at least two years, though most risk managers keep them on file for at least five years because the statute of limitations on problems related to medical devices is at least this long. The Safe Medical Devices Act also applies to devices that are permanently implantable or life-sustaining and designed to be used outside of the medical facilities (e.g., pacemakers). In order to track these devices, the final distributor is responsible for sending identifying information about the user to the manufacturer.

Reusable single use devices
The Food and Drug Administration (FDA) rules related to single-use devices are outlined in the publication, "Guidance on Enforcement Priorities for Single-Use Devices Reprocessed by Third Parties and Hospitals." According to these policies, for instance, any company that reprocesses a single-use device must register itself with the FDA and must file a list of the devices to be reprocessed. In addition, the act specifies that any hospitals or independent reprocessors must follow the same device tracking strictures as the manufacturers. According to the FDA, whenever certain repairs, modifications, or recalls are made with the intent of reducing a risk to the health of the patient, a report must be filed. In addition, the FDA has established certain quality system regulations, which cover the oversight of materials and techniques used in the design, production, packaging, labeling, storage, and use of these devices. With respect to labeling, the FDA requires that a device's package should include the product's name, manufacturer, point of origin, and directions for use. For risk managers, all of these rules necessitate a great degree of oversight.

Mammography Quality Standards Act of 1992

The Mammography Quality Standards Act of 1992 (MQSA), amended in the Mammography Quality Standards Reauthorization Acts of 1998 and 2004, was intended to improve the quality of mammography in the United States. It established specific training and education standards for radiological technicians, medical physicists, and physicians. It also mandated that facilities be annually accredited either by the FDA or by an FDA-approved body. The act also standardized the protocol for reporting the results of a mammogram to the patient and to the referring healthcare provider. The act outlined the protocols for developing and implementing quality assurance and quality control programs, and mandated specific equipment testing and maintenance procedures. All of these rules are available for risk managers in a single location, the MQSA guidance publication issued by the FDA.

Newborns' and Mothers' Health Protection Act of 1996

The Newborns' and Mothers' Health Protection Act of 1996 was intended to ensure that new mothers and newborns receive adequate healthcare. The act was issued because of a widespread perception that many medical facilities were forcing new mothers to leave the hospital too early. The act applies to obstetricians, group health plans, and any other facilities that provide obstetrical services. The general rule is that a mother and her newborn must receive covered hospital benefits for at least 48 hours after a vaginal delivery or 96 hours after a cesarean section. However, the mother and newborn may be discharged earlier if the mother agrees. In some cases, state laws may supersede this federal act, but only if they do not diminish the minimum allowable covered stay.

National Organ Transplant Act of 1984

The National Organ Transplant Act of 1984 created a nationwide system for collecting and distributing organs for transplant. Since the passage of this law, the Organ Procurement Transplant Network (OPTN) has operated as a collaboration between the United Network for Organ Sharing and the Division of Transplantation of the Health Resources and Services Administration. The National Organ and Tissue Donation Initiative is another organization that contributes to this program. These various groups have worked to improve oversight of the transplantation process, develop specific performance criteria, and promote accountability. To be a member of the OPTN, a hospital needs to establish working agreements with an organ procurement organization, a tissue bank, and an eye bank, under which the hospital will provide notification whenever a patient is about to die or has just died. The hospital is not responsible for determining whether the deceased is a suitable donor: this judgment should be made by the organ procurement organization. Members of the OPTN should also inform potential donors and their families about the options for donation. Participation in OPTN is a condition of participation in Medicare for many facilities.

CLIA of 1988

The Clinical Laboratory Improvement Amendments of 1988 (CLIA) defined quality standards for clinical laboratories. Previous to the enactment of these amendments, there was widespread disorganization in laboratories. The law has changed over time, so risk managers should refer to the website of the Division of Laboratory Systems, a part of the Centers for Disease Control and Prevention. The law distinguishes three covered test categories: waived complexity, moderate complexity, and high complexity. The requirements are more onerous for more complex tests. Laboratories are required to pay a fee and complete a certification process to enroll in the CLIA program.

Human research subjects

The most important document related to research on people is the Protection of Human Subjects regulations. According to this document, an institutional review board (IRB) must examine any proposed research before it may be undertaken. Once research has been approved by the IRB, it may still need to be reviewed and approved by officials from the sponsoring institution. The research group must receive informed consent from any participants. To be complete, the consent must include the following eight components: description of the research, explication of the purpose and anticipated length of the study, a summary of the predictable risks or discomforts, explanation of the anticipated benefits of the research, description of any alternative procedures that are available, the details of the confidentiality agreement, identification of the contact individual, and an assertion that participation is voluntary and that the subject has not been coerced. If the research involves a greater-than-minimal risk, the informed consent should include an explanation of the compensation policy in the event the participant becomes injured. This consent must be signed by the subject or by his or her authorized legal representative.

Medicare regulations for long-term care facilities

Long-term care facilities have received a great deal of attention from the office of the Inspector General in recent years. In particular, the government has been concerned about Medicare billing irregularities in these facilities. To maintain Medicare funding, long-term care facilities must develop specific initiatives to improve the general level of care, decrease the incidence of malnutrition and bed sores, and make sure that all the rights patients deserve are supported in practice. Specifically, patients have the rights to information about their health, medical benefits, and the costs of treatment; access to a physician; copies of their medical records; participation in treatment decisions (including the right of refusal and the right to prepare advance directives); freedom from unnecessary psychoactive drugs and physical restraints; and the freedom to file formal complaints when these rights have been violated.

Life Safety Code

The Life Safety Code is a set of fire safety requirements that were adopted by the Centers for Medicare and Medicaid Services after being drafted by the National Fire Protection Association. Unless they are granted a waiver, facilities that receive Medicare funds are required to comply with the Life Safety Code. The code mainly addresses issues like emergency alarm systems, emergency lighting, and program waivers. The Life Safety Code also has specific regulations related to hospices and ambulatory surgery centers. Facilities are required to complete a basic building information form, which should include the current floor plans for any part of the building that provides the designated patient or resident services. For the most part, compliance with the Life Safety Code will be the responsibility of the facility's engineers and safety officers, but the risk manager will no doubt be involved in the process as well because the Life Safety Code is essentially a document of risk management.

Nuclear Regulatory Commission

The Nuclear Regulatory Commission (NRC) was established in 1954 as part of the Atomic Energy Act. This body is responsible for overseeing the handling, storage, and use of radioactive substances. The purview of the NRC includes the use of these substances in the medical field in the following instances: research with human subjects; administration of palliative or therapeutic doses to specific tissues or anatomical areas; and during radioactive uptake, dilution, excretion, imaging, or local diagnostic clinical or research procedures. Whenever an error occurs during the administration of a nuclear by-product, it must be reported within 15 days. Also, the Nuclear Regulatory Commission mandates a long series of staff training exercises, and levies penalties for organizations that do not comply. The NRC also requires facilities to maintain a quality management program. The regulations of the NRC are most important to those risk managers whose facilities handle a great deal of radioactive materials, but every risk manager should be somewhat conversant with these regulations because failure to comply can result in the loss of an NRC license.

National Elder Abuse Incidence Study

The National Elder Abuse Incidence Study was somewhat limited in its scope because it only addressed elder abuse in homes. In other words, the abuse of elders in medical facilities and nursing homes was not considered. Elder abuse can include abduction by family members; physical, sexual, or emotional abuse; abandonment; neglect; and financial exploitation. There are a number of mandatory reporting requirements related to elder abuse, and risk managers must be sure that they comply with these. Some of these reporting requirements were created by individual institutions, while others derive from state law. There are also a number of elder abuse-related exceptions to other reporting requirements. For instance, some of the documents related to substance abuse treatment programs may be treated according to different confidentiality standards in cases of suspected elder or child abuse.

Risk management implications of Medicare

Medicare has specific implications for risk management. It is the largest health insurance program in the United States, and is administered by the Centers for Medicare and Medicaid Services (CMS) of the Department of Health and Human Services. Medicare is divided into two parts. Part A, hospital insurance, provides coverage for inpatient hospital services, home healthcare, hospice care, and brief stays in skilled nursing facilities. Part B, supplementary medical insurance, offers coverage for ambulance trips, durable medical equipment, physician services, outpatient services, and some elements of home healthcare. Payments made as part of the Medicare system are transacted by private companies, known as carriers, which are designated by the CMS. The responsibility for overseeing Medicare lies with the CMS in general, although healthcare facilities and financial intermediaries are certified by state licensing and regulatory agencies.

Risk management implications of Medicaid

Medicaid has specific implications for risk management. At present, there are 25 categories of people who may be eligible for Medicaid coverage. Some of these are the disabled, children, and pregnant women. Medicaid programs are administered by the states, and indeed each state has a great deal of freedom with regard to how the programs are organized, how rates are set, and how eligibility standards are arranged. Consequently, a risk manager must be familiar with the particular Medicaid program in his or her state. There are currently more than 40 million people covered under Medicaid. Many of these are recipients of Medicare who have limited economic resources and have been granted supplemental coverage under Medicaid for specific supplies or services.

Risk management implications of ERISA

The Employee Retirement Income Security Act of 1974 (ERISA) is of particular interest to risk managers who deal with employee benefit or managed care programs. The main consequence of this act has been a decrease in the number of successful lawsuits by plaintiffs who feel that they are owed money according to state laws guaranteeing plan benefits. It should be noted by risk managers that ERISA does not give healthcare providers the right to deny service. In other words, the provisions of the Emergency Medical Treatment and Leave Act (EMTALA) supersede those of ERISA with regards to service provision, if not the source of payment. Whenever the denial of treatment is the result of decisions made by the managed care plan or employee benefit program, the healthcare institution should collect extensive records because of the likelihood of litigation. Moreover, the facility should always tell the patient why service has been denied, and should outline alternative treatments that may be available.

Tort reform

During the 1970s, the amount of professional malpractice litigation in the United States ballooned, which placed an onerous burden on risk managers. One effort to control these law suits has been tort reform, which has mostly been enacted at the state level. In particular, California's Medical Injury Compensation Reform Act, or MICRA, has been a model for state reforms. This act was passed in 1975, and it took direct steps to combat the damage a medical facility could suffer as a result of malpractice suits. To begin with, MICRA established a $250,000 cap for noneconomic damages, often referred to as "pain and suffering." The act also allowed liable facilities to repay their damages over time, which made it easier for them to endure heavy losses. The act also declared that juries are allowed to learn about alternative sources of compensation for plaintiffs so that the entire financial burden does not fall on the medical facility. Finally, MICRA put a cap on the rates of attorney's contingency fees.

Professional practice acts

The professional practice acts are used to determine whether a practitioner has performed an action outside of his or her scope of practice. The professional practice acts vary by state. It is very important for a risk manager to be familiar with the professional practice acts, as these often decide whether a loss will be covered by insurance. In addition, malpractice suits often hinge on the court's definition of scope of practice. The state professional practice acts will define the scope of practice and the authority for oversight. They are the foundation of the facility's standards of care. Moreover, a risk manager will refer to the professional practice acts during the development of new treatments, so that these do not overstep the appropriate boundaries of professional practice.

Effects of case law on risk management

Case law has specific effects on risk management. When the courts make rulings that affect case law, these rulings have the strength of legislation. However, advances in case law may not receive the same attention as new laws, so it is especially important for risk managers to be vigilant about keeping abreast of changes. Fortunately, risk managers have a number of resources to consult, including judicial Web pages, the publications of the American Society for Healthcare Risk Management, and regulatory updates put out by the state healthcare organizations. Typically, the risk manager is responsible for drafting summaries of relevant case laws, and distributing these summaries to the staff. In particular, a risk manager needs to do a good job of informing employees about how changes in case law affect their work.

Ethical medical research

The seminal document of medical research ethics is the Belmont Report issued by the National Commission for the Protection of Human Subjects in Biomedical and Behavioral Research in 1979. This report listed three essential ethical characteristics for research on human subjects: justice, beneficence, and respect for persons. Justice is defined as an equitable distribution of both the rewards and the burdens of research. Beneficence is the moral imperative to make research both as positive in its effects and as minimal in its risks as possible. The report defines respect for persons as acknowledgment of the individual dignity and autonomy of each person, as well as concern and special treatment for vulnerable populations, whether the very young, the very old, or the ill.

Institutional review boards for medical research

There are a number of institutional review boards whose mission is to ensure that research is conducted according to ethical standards. Institutional review boards also monitor issues related to informed consent, subject selection, and confidentiality. Institutional review boards identify the risks of research and try to ensure that those risks will be minimized as much as possible. Institutional review boards require research facilities to define the intended and probable benefits of the research, and to demonstrate that the potential rewards outweigh any attendant risk. Institutional review boards ensure that research subjects are provided with adequate information about the research, both in terms of the anticipated benefits and the risks. Research participants should have the opportunity to agree or decline to participate in the research, and they should not feel subject to any threat of reprisal or coercion. Finally, institutional review boards establish programs for periodic review. These organizations have an array of assessments for measuring the performance and ethical record of active researchers.

Ethics of gene or recombinant DNA research

Whenever research requires the use of federally funded recombinant DNA or gene therapy, it must be reviewed by the Institutional Biosafety Committee and the Recombinant DNA Advisory Committee of the Office of Biotechnology Activities. Naturally, there is a great deal of interest in the ethical implications of gene manipulation. Risk managers should periodically review their institution's policies and procedures, as well as their record of compliance with the relevant institutional review boards. The risk manager should ensure that the institution has specific policies in place to promote compliance with the safety criteria prioritized by the institutional review boards. There is also a greater risk of costly litigation for research companies that perform gene or recombinant DNA research. These companies should take professional, general liability, or directors' and officers' insurance to cover this risk.

Ethical issues related to medical record privacy

There are a number of ethical issues related to medical record privacy. To begin with, the common rule asserts that institutional review boards are responsible for monitoring the steps being taken by research institutions to protect the confidentiality of subjects. The Health Insurance Portability and Accountability Act established a number of requirements in 2003 for the handling of protected health information (PHI). The provisions of the act are enforced by the federal Department of Health and Human Services. Institutions are allowed to use or disclose PHI only under the following specific circumstances: when a privacy board or institutional review board has approved a waiver of the confidentiality requirements; when the data is reviewed by a researcher preparatory to research, and the researcher does not remove the data from the premises; when the institution has received authorization from the research subject to use the protected health information; or when there is a data use agreement between the institution and the researcher to transmit a limited data set. In this last case, the patient information must not be transmitted in a form that permits facial identification.

Response to false identification or possession of illegal drugs

There are a number of reasons why a patient at a healthcare facility might present false identification: to obtain medication, to commit Medicare fraud, or to avoid violations of his or her privacy. Whatever the reason, the healthcare facility is required to act immediately when a false presentation is discovered. In most states, the facility is required to notify the state health department. However, the presentation of false identification is never grounds for denial of service by a healthcare facility. The mandates of the Emergency Medical Treatment and Leave Act still apply in cases of false presentation. If a patient is found to be in possession of illegal drugs, however, the facility may be required to report the patient to law enforcement, in which case he or she may be removed from the facility. Many healthcare facilities conduct unscheduled tests for illegal drugs among the inpatient population, not only because the possession of these drugs may constitute a violation of the law, but because their use may be counterproductive to the treatment protocol.

Authorization for use and disclosure of PHI for research

According to the Health Insurance Portability and Accountability Act, the protected health information (PHI) of deceased individuals is subject to the same restrictions as the PHI of living. It should be noted, however, that if all identifiers have been removed from the information, it is not considered PHI. In order for information to be de-identified, all of the following must be removed: names; geographical subdivisions smaller than a state (the first three digits of the ZIP Code are permitted); dates (except year) for any subjects younger than 90; telephone numbers; email addresses; fax numbers; Social Security numbers; medical record numbers; account numbers; certificate or license numbers; health plan beneficiary numbers; vehicle identifiers and serial numbers (including license plates); device identifiers and serial numbers; URLs; Internet protocol addresses; biometric identifiers (e.g. voice prints, fingerprints); boldface photographs or any equivalent damages; and any other unique identifying characteristic, number, or code.

There are specific requirements for a valid authorization for the use of protected health information (PHI) in research. To begin with, the research institution must describe what PHI will be used or disclosed, as well as the person or class of persons who will use or have access to the protected health information. The research institution also needs to indicate how the information will be used. Finally, the research institution must indicate whether there is a possibility of redisclosure, and must give an expiration date, the signature and date of the subject, and an explicit right to revoke. There are a few common exceptions from the authorization requirements. For instance, the authorization requirements may be waived if there is no more than a minimal risk to the privacy of the subject, or if the research institution provides assurance that protected health information will not be reused or disclosed except when required by the law or the needs of the research itself. A waiver may also be granted if the research could not be conducted either without the waiver or without the personal health information.

Patient Self-Determination Act of 1990

The Patient Self-Determination Act of 1990 requires federally funded healthcare providers to give patients the right to make decisions about their healthcare. For instance, patients should have the right to accept or refuse treatment, as well as to create living wills and durable powers of attorney (commonly grouped under the heading of advance directives). When a patient is admitted, the facility must provide a set of written information outlining the patient's rights to make healthcare decisions. The constitutional right to patient self-determination was explained by the Supreme Court as emanating from the due process clause of the 14th Amendment. In situations where a patient is unable to provide informed consent, his or her rights of self-determination are to be exercised by a surrogate. This is another reason why it is important for patients to grant a durable power of attorney to the person whom they would wish to make decisions should they become incapacitated.

Joint Commission's sentinel event policy

The Joint Commission's sentinel event policy seeks to promote habitual reporting so that accurate statistics about adverse events can be created. Any event that has an adverse effect on a patient must be reported. However, facilities are not required to report the following events: unexpected death or major permanent loss of function unrelated to the natural course of the patient's illness or underlying condition; unexpected death of a full-term infant; discharge of an infant to the wrong family; rape; suicide of any person receiving care, treatment, or services in a staffed around-the-clock care setting or within 72 hours of discharge; abduction of any person receiving care, treatment, or services; hemolytic transfusion reaction involving the administration of blood or blood products with major blood group incompatibilities; surgery on the wrong patient or body part; severe neonatal hyperbilirubinemia; prolonged fluoroscopy with a cumulative dose greater than 1500 rads to a single field or any delivery of radiotherapy to the wrong body region or greater than 25 percent above the planned radiotherapy dose; or the unintended retention of a foreign object in a person after surgery or another medical procedure.

Handling sentinel events that are not self-reported

The Joint Commission typically receives reports of sentinel events from medical facilities, but in some cases the report is made by an employee, the media, a patient, or a patient's family member. If the event is not subject to the mandatory reporting requirements, the Joint Commission's response will not be affected by the source of the report. In other words, the time frame within which the event will be reviewed and handled will not be changed. The Joint Commission strives to create an atmosphere in which facilities will feel comfortable self-reporting, but it is aware that there are many reasons why a sentinel event may go unreported. The Joint Commission therefore makes it possible for sentinel event reports to be made anonymously, so long as the event is not subject to the mandatory reporting requirements.

Joint Commission response to sentinel events

The Joint Commission response to a sentinel event is organized according to a standard protocol. To begin with, the Joint Commission will make a preliminary judgment as to whether the event is indeed a reviewable sentinel event. Then, the medical facility at which the event occurred will be required to prepare a complete root cause analysis (RCA) and action plan within 45 days of the date of the event or the date on which the organization became aware of the event. The root cause analysis and action plan also must be submitted within 45 calendar days of the sentinel event's occurrence. The root cause analysis and action must meet the Joint Commission's standard for credibility and comprehensiveness.

Advantages of reporting sentinel events to the Joint Commission

There are several advantages to reporting sentinel events to the Joint Commission. To begin with, reporting enables the facility to confer with the Joint Commission during the preparation of the root cause analysis and action plan. Reporting helps the organization learn more about the prevalence and possible causes of the sentinel event. It may enable the organization to learn more about how to prevent similar events from happening in the future. The facility will also receive a public relations boost from reporting because this indicates that the facility is proactive about dealing with errors and adverse events. The Joint Commission makes every effort to keep sentinel event reports confidential. To this end, healthcare organizations are discouraged from including patient or employee identification in reports. All copies of both the root cause analysis and the action plan will be either returned to the facility or destroyed by the Joint Commission.

Submission of the root cause analysis and action plan to the Joint Commission

There are five acceptable protocols for submitting a root cause analysis and action plan to the Joint Commission. First, the organization may present a root cause analysis and a set of action plan documents to the headquarters of the Joint Commission for review. The organization must then take the documents back on the same day. Another option is for a trained surveyor to perform a visit in situ, during which he or she will review the root cause analysis and action plan. It is also permissible for the trained surveyor to visit the site and review the root cause analysis and findings, even if he or she does not specifically examine the root cause analysis documents, so long as there is also a review of the relevant information and a series of informative interviews. The surveyor may also perform a standards-based survey that considers the care, treatment, and services of the patient as well as the management functions of the organization insofar as they relate to the sentinel event being reviewed. Finally, the organization may indicate that it meets the given criteria related to the risk of waiving legal protection for root cause information shared with the Joint Commission, so long as the trained surveyor conducts an inspection on site, interviews the staff, and collects information about how the organization responds to sentinel events.

Reporting systems administered by the FDA

The Food and Drug Administration manages several reporting systems, including MedWatch Form 3500, the Manufacturers and User Facility Device Experience (MAUDE) database, Adverse Event Reporting System, and Vaccine Adverse Event Reporting System. MedWatch Form 3500 was mandated by the Dietary Supplement and Nonprescription Drug Consumer Protection Act of 2006; it requires medical organizations to report adverse events related to dietary supplements. The MAUDE database is a record of adverse events related to medical devices. It was mandated by the Safe Medical Devices Act of 1990. Manufacturers, importers, and end users are all required to submit these reports. The Adverse Event Reporting System (AERS) is a collection of adverse event reports subsequent to approved drugs. The Vaccine Adverse Event Reporting System (VAERS) is a cooperative activity of the Food and Drug Administration and the Centers for Disease Control. VAERS is a record of adverse events that occur subsequent to the administration of a vaccine.

Systems for reporting medical errors

There are a number of systems for reporting medical errors. The Institute for Safe Medication Practices and United States Pharmacopeia administer the Medication Error Reporting program, which generates a record of anonymous information from physicians, nurses, and pharmacists. The intention of this database is to solve common problems. The National Coordinating Council for Medication Error Reporting and Prevention created a medication error index in 1996. This index places medication errors in one of nine categories, depending on the severity of the outcome.

The Medical Event Reporting System—Transfusion Medicine is administered by Columbia University. It is a repository of adverse events, errors, and near misses related to blood transfusions. Reports are made anonymously, and participants are given access to the entire database. The Intensive Care Unit Safety Reporting System (ICUSRS) is a collaboration between Johns Hopkins University and the Society for Critical Care Medicine; it is an example of the burgeoning number of adverse event reporting systems covering subspecialties. The Pittsburgh Regional Healthcare Initiative began as an informal collaboration between business leaders and healthcare executives, but has become a leading voice in the evolution of healthcare quality management. Finally, the Patient Safety Reporting System, which is overseen by the United States Department of Veterans Affairs, keeps a record of all the medical errors that occur within the VA.

National Quality Forum's *Standardizing a Patient Safety Taxonomy* and the Joint Commission's recommendations for protection of sensitive information

The National Quality Forum in 2006 released a report entitled *Standardizing a Patient Safety Taxonomy*, in which the NQF advanced a comprehensive system for classifying data about patient safety. The Patient Safety Event Taxonomy (PSET) is a problem-solving tool for hospital administrators and healthcare practitioners alike. It is expected that the use of this taxonomy will improve the quality of service and the ability of healthcare facilities to meet challenges. With respect to sensitive information, the Joint Commission has devised methods for organizations to provide sentinel event and adverse event reports without becoming subject to legal orders for discovery. This enables the healthcare facility to mount an appropriate defense against legal challenges without compromising the standard of reporting.

Patient Safety and Quality Improvement Act of 2005

The Patient Safety and Quality Improvement Act of 2005 created a standard framework for the collection and protection of records related to patient safety. This act created a nationwide database of medical errors. In addition, the act enabled the creation of patient safety organizations (PSOs), which must be approved by the Secretary of the US Department of Health and Human Services. The Patient Safety and Quality Improvement Act of 2005 also mandated confidentiality restrictions for particular patient safety work products collected under a patient safety evaluation system. PSOs are certified by the Department of Health and Human Services. The interactions of the Patient Safety and Quality Improvement Act and similar state laws vary by jurisdiction, so risk managers should evaluate how these laws are enforced in their area.

Healthcare Operations

Medical record

A medical record must include some basic components. The following are essential components of a medical record: admission, identification, or face sheet; vital signs and graphics sheet; medical, surgical, and health history and physical condition; problem list; medication record; progress notes; physicians' orders; discharge notes; and any authorization forms. Authorization forms may include any consent forms for admission, treatment, surgery, or the release of medical records. The medical record may also include any of the following: non-stress test report, fetal monitoring strip, labor and delivery record, recovery room record, anesthesia record, transfer record, autopsy report, consultation report, operative report, emergency department record, lab report, imaging and X-ray report, and electrocardiogram. In addition, the following types of document will often be relevant to the work of a risk manager: financial records, employee health records, billing records, OSHA records, radiology films, accreditation and other inspection reports, contracts, incidence and occurrence reports, and insurance policies.

Medical documentation

Medical documentation is the essential record keeping related to the provision of medical services. Documents are an essential part of the legal record, and establish a basis for the service provider's reimbursement. Documents are also important because they are a chronological record of the care provided to the patient, and are therefore instrumental in the planning and evaluation of treatment protocols. An effective documentation system improves communication between service providers and thereby improves the quality and continuity of care. Medical documentation ensures that a facility is providing an appropriate level of care, as well as that the facility is meeting the appropriate standard of care. In order for medical documentation to fulfill all of these requirements, it must be clear, comprehensive, and accessible to stakeholders.

Medical documentation and accreditation, licensure, and regulatory requirements

There are a number of external authorities that make requirements with respect to medical documentation. Perhaps the most important of these is the Health Insurance Portability and Accountability Act, which establishes particular rules for the confidentiality of certain documents, known collectively as protected health information (PHI). The federal Centers for Medicare and Medicaid Services (CMS) mandates the following pieces of information: physical examination records, admitting diagnosis, results of clinical evaluation, any records related to complications or adverse reactions to medication, any required informed consent forms, related practitioner's orders, and a discharge summary and final diagnosis. There are also a number of documentation requirements made by professional advancement organizations, among them the American Nurses Association, American Medical Association, Health Insurance Association of America, Health Information Management Systems Society, and American Health Information Management System. Finally, the Joint Commission has established a number of standards for medical record keeping, among them that facilities maintain complete and accurate records for all patients, that the record explains in detail any operations or use of sedation, and that the record include any medications administered and diagnoses made.

Essential charting components

The Joint Commission Standards for essential charting components, as outlined in Standard IM 6.20, are quite detailed. According to these standards, a medical record must contain the following: description of the emergency care, treatment, and services provided before arrival at the facility; documentation and assessment findings; conclusions made from physical examination and medical history; diagnosis, diagnostic impression, or conditions; reasons for admission, treatment, or services; goals of the treatment plan; diagnostic and therapeutic orders; diagnostic and therapeutic procedures, tests, and results; authorized progress notes; plan of care revisions; relevant observations; response to treatment; allergies to foods and medications; medications used or prescribed; consultation reports; and any conditions or diagnoses established during the course of care, treatment, and services. Moreover, the medical record should contain the following demographic information: patient's name, gender, address, date of birth, and authorized representative; legal status; known advance directives; informed consent patient care; and records of communication. Finally, patients who are receiving continuous ambulatory care should have the following information included in their medical record: significant medical diagnoses and conditions; operative and invasive procedures; adverse and allergic drug reactions; and any long-term medications, including herbal and over-the-counter medications.

Documentation models

In charting by exception, only information that deviates from the norm is recorded. This method was devised to reduce the amount of redundant information in the medical record, but it has largely been abandoned because it presents the medical record as a litany of errors and adverse events. In addition, there is evidence that charting by exception tends to exclude useful information, as for instance the evolution of the patient's condition. In narrative charting, on the other hand, a chronological record is kept of the patient's condition, treatment, and response. Too often, however, these notes are excessively long and full of irrelevancies. In assessment-intervention-response (AIR) documentation, the medical record is organized as a narrative, but with emphasis on certain major events. Flowsheets are used to record dates, times, and interventions; these documents are organized in a grid formation. A checklist is simply a list of the tasks that must be completed with respect to patient care.

Focus charting emphasizes major changes and events. It is most appropriate, then, for acute care and situations in which the same treatment protocols are enacted frequently. The problem-oriented medical record system, otherwise known as POMR, is also used frequently in acute care: it uses a series of progress notes to describe particular patient events and problems. The problem, interventions, and evaluations of interventions (PIE) approach uses the patient's problems as the organizing principle and makes the plan of care an important part of the nurses' progress notes. FACT stands for flowsheets, assessment, concise, and timely: it is a system that advocates the use of targeted, succinct, and immediate flowsheets. Once again, this system was devised to eliminate redundancies and irrelevancies in the medical record. The core approach is primarily used in long-term and acute care facilities, where it emphasizes the process of nursing. The critical pathway approach organizes the record as progress along a specific timeline, with major categories like diet, activities, treatments, activities, and discharge planning.

One of the most popular documentation models is known by the acronym SOAP, for subjective, objective, assessment, and plan. (Occasionally, the model is known as SOAPIER, with the extra letters standing for interventions, evaluations, and revision.) This model is used in all sorts of care settings: ambulatory, home care, acute care, and long-term care. This model is used specifically for the progress notes section of the medical record. The SOAP model is good for creating a holistic account of the patient's trouble, and easily identifying the goals and methods of treatment. The model makes it easier for professionals in different areas to communicate with one another, and establishes a standard system for organizing and describing problems. However, the SOAP model must be taught to everyone, and requires the full commitment of the entire staff. In addition, the model must be fulfilled in its totality, or else the organizational improvements are lost. The SOAP model can be somewhat time-consuming relative to other documentation models, and therefore may be more subject to errors by staff members.

Correcting medical record errors

There are specific protocols for correcting errors in the medical record. The staff member should draw a single line through the entry, place his or her initials or signature and the date next to the error, and write the correction above the error. If there is not enough space for the correction on the document, the correction should be made at the relevant place on the record, whether in the progress notes or the nursing notes. Employees should not make any corrections that hide the original error, as for instance by whiting out or erasing. It is important that the record contain evidence of the error as well as of the correction. Otherwise, the medical care facility may be accused of tampering with records in order to appear less culpable.

Hearsay and telephone conversations in medical records

There are special protocols for handling hearsay and telephone conversations with respect to medical records. Hearsay is defined as statements made by persons other than the author of the medical record. These statements should not be written down as if they were fact. The record should contain a description of the source of the information, and the information itself should be placed within quotation marks. Telephone calls are another source of trouble in medical records because there is often no way to verify the identity of the recipient of information. A medical facility should have an established protocol for who is allowed to dispense information over the phone, as well as what types of information may be disclosed. The medical record should include the caller, the date, the time, and the reason for the call. After the call, the record should include a description of the response to the call as well.

Physician notifications in medical records

Medical records should include detailed information regarding every contact with a physician. The record should include the date and time of the contact as well as its content. With regard to the latter, the conversation should include a description of the patient's signs and symptoms, and the results of any laboratory evaluations. The physician's response should be recorded also. If the medical record indicates that the patient has attempted to get in touch with the physician but the physician has taken too long to respond, the nurse should follow the institution's chain of command and contact the next appropriate professional. Each institution should establish its own standards for the duration within which a physician should respond to a request.

Countersignatures, abbreviations, and authentication in medical records

A countersignature indicates that the healthcare provider has not only read and signed the order, but that he or she endorses the given treatment protocol. A healthcare provider who signs a medical record is thereby becoming responsible for the information contained in that entry. This is often true of admission notes, history and physical records, operative notes, and discharge summaries, so it is important for the healthcare provider to read the documents carefully before signing. When the facility uses an electronic system of record keeping, the healthcare provider should use an electronic signature. Medical records should only use abbreviations in situations that have been pre-approved. Because of the high risk of error when abbreviations are used, the Joint Commission and the Institute for Safe Medication Practices have published lists of abbreviations that should not be employed. Finally, facilities should follow special protocols to ensure that only authorized people contribute to records. Specifically, all entries should contain a date, time, and signature of the author.

Termination of care records

It is especially important for there to be comprehensive and accurate records related to the termination of care because this event is often an occasion for litigation or dispute. When a medical facility elects to suspend or terminate treatment, the standard protocol is first to deliver the message orally, and then to follow that with a written directive. It is typical for the written notice to include a description of the ongoing care the patient should receive over a certain interval, usually the next 30 days. This description of continuing care should include all of the necessary prescriptions, complete with refill orders. In addition, it is typical for the written report provided to the patient to include a list of referrals, or physicians in similar areas who could also provide service to the patient.

Appropriate terminology and legibility in medical records

Medical records should be written clearly and simply. A standard terminology should be used to avoid confusion. For instance, a medical record should not use terms that indicate an accident has happened unless this meaning is intended. A medical record should not suggest that something that occurred was unintended or unexpected unless it truly was so. Moreover, a medical record should not include vague or unclear language, as this sort of language can be manipulated by defense attorneys to suggest doubt. Perhaps most importantly, medical staff should be careful to avoid assigning or suggesting error by a coworker. The medical record should not contain blame or apologies for errors during service provision. It is acceptable for the record to indicate empathy when appropriate. The record should not include any speculation or uninformed opinion. Any differences of opinion between medical staff should be discussed privately and not in the records. Finally, the medical record must be legible at all times. There have been several cases in which illegible records have led to a settlement against the facility.

Documenting medical errors

A medical record may be introduced as evidence in a trial, so it is very important that errors be documented according to a certain protocol. However, the medical record does not need to include a mention or a description of the incident report or the actions of the risk management department. The medical record should include a description of the incident and how it was resolved. When a medical professional needs to document an error, he or she should categorize the error according to the terminology approved by the organization. The record should include the actual time of the event, as well as what happened and who was immediately notified. The medical record should not refer to the event as a "medical error," but should focus on documenting the objective elements of the event. The medical record should also describe the response to the event and the implemented treatment plan. Finally, the medical record should describe the disclosure discussion, as this will preclude allegations of a cover-up.

Record retention

The following statutes and bodies have requirements for the length of time a record should be retained: Joint Commission, the Centers for Medicare and Medicaid Services, the Occupational Safety and Health Administration, the Public Health Services Act, the National Childhood Vaccine Injury Act, and the National Commission on Correctional Healthcare for Health Services in Jails and Prisons. The risk management department must be familiar with the record retention requirements for each of these, as well as those imposed by the federal reimbursement requirements and the policies of the institution itself. There are some basic guidelines for record retention. Any records related to an ongoing investigation should be retained. Patient health information should only be disposed of according to a clear and written schedule. In most organizations, medical records are kept in a single location, but whenever it is necessary to keep some records elsewhere, the retention protocol should include specific guidelines for these locations. Before going into effect, the retention policy should receive the approval of the organization's legal counsel, chief executive officer, health information manager, and medical staff.

Release of records

Medical records should only be released in accordance with the regulations of the federal and state governments and the organization itself. The organization's policy for record release should indicate which parties are eligible to request copies of the medical record. The policy should also name those parties who are authorized to release records, as well as those parties to whom records may be released. The policy should describe how the access to medical records will be assessed and documented, and how sensitive information will be protected. When the medical facility fails to follow the proper procedures for the release of information, there may be severe legal consequences. Also, the organization should maintain a strict definition of the legal health record. The definition advanced by the American Health Information Management Association is that the legal health record is synonymous with the health facility's business record. It is this record which will be disclosed upon request.

Ownership of records and medical record audits

The ownership arrangement of medical records is somewhat tricky because the patient owns the information contained in the record and the healthcare facility owns the record itself. With some variation from state to state, the patient has the right to request information from the record, but the healthcare facility has the right to retain a physical copy of the record. These days, it is most common for disputes about the ownership of records to emerge from mergers and acquisitions. One way to ensure that the record-keeping process is orderly and legal is to conduct regular audits. An audit should address certain key questions, as for instance whether the reason for the patient encounter has been recorded, and whether the record clearly explains the resulting course of treatment. The audit should also ascertain whether records contain enough information to justify the medical decisions, and whether the documentation practices are in accordance with all applicable requirements.

Medical records and liability exposure

The most important aspect of medical record-keeping is creating a set of documents that will facilitate adequate patient care. However, it is also crucial for medical records to prevent the organization from suffering unnecessary liability exposure. To this end, the organization should strive to avoid vague or contradictory statements in the record. Whenever there are indications of disagreement or conflict between practitioners, the record should resolve these issues. The record can be challenged if there are obvious omissions, as for instance when the order for a test is indicated but the results are not in the record. A medical record should never be corrected in a manner that suggests the error was being removed. This is why white-out and erasers should never be used on a medical record. The medical record should be free of ambiguous language. Finally, the medical record must always contain any informed consent or patient education documentation related to the case.

Protecting privileged information and forensic documentation examination

There are some medical documents that are not subject to discovery during legal proceedings. However, the precise types of documents that are privileged vary from state to state. The risk manager should be aware of the documents that are confidential, privileged, or protected by attorney-client privilege in his or her state. In healthcare, the following types of documents may be privileged: incident reports, incident investigations, peer review proceedings, root cause analyses, corrective action plans, risk and quality management committee records, and corrective action plans. There are also situations in which a privileged document may become subject to discovery, as for instance when the healthcare facility shares it with a third party.

Techniques of forensic documentation examination

When medical documents are a part of legal proceedings, investigators have a battery of forensic examination techniques at their disposal. For instance, investigators may use a variety of techniques for ink analysis when there is a suspicion that the document has been altered. These techniques are able to distinguish between the types of ink used to mark a document. Infrared technology can also be used to identify ink types, though it is not capable of demonstrating that inks are the same. However, unlike other ink analysis techniques, infrared examination does not damage the document. Forensic examiners will also look for any relevant date markers which can be used to identify when a document was produced by a printer or copy machine. In the technique called electrostatic detection, investigators are able to identify residual impressions on the pages underneath an altered document. Finally, there are certified handwriting analysts who are capable of distinguishing the origins of even the smallest markings on a medical record. However, when handwriting analysis is to be performed, the risk manager must be able to demonstrate the chain of custody for the evidence throughout the process, to prevent allegations of tampering.

Preparation of documentation before legal action

When a risk manager expects legal action, he or she should be sure to abide by the claim reporting procedures that have been established by the organization. The risk manager should ensure that all the essential records are secure, and that copies of these records have only been released in response to a written request. When copies of a medical record are released, the risk manager should ensure that only the pertinent parts of the record are released. The risk manager should not allow a medical record to be altered once it has been requested and a copy has been released. There are explicit rules related to documentation in the Federal Rules of Civil Procedure (FRCP). Although many medical professional liability cases are adjudicated in state court, these courts mostly abide by a close facsimile of the FRCP.

Electronic recordkeeping and CPOE

Increasingly, medical facilities in the United States are keeping electronic records of their patients. There are all sorts of advantages to using electronic records: greater accessibility, elimination of redundant tests, and compilation of a patient's entire medical record. However, the transition to electronic records is a tricky process that creates the opportunity for error. In order for electronic recordkeeping to work, the staff must be involved in the development of the program and must be trained comprehensively once the program has been implemented. Moreover, there needs to be a clear and easy protocol for making corrections to the medical record. Computerized physician order entry (CPOE) systems, meanwhile, are electronic systems specifically for doctor's orders. Many of the facilities that have implemented CPOE report that it has drastically reduced transcription errors. A further concern is that medical records may be accessed by hackers and other malefactors, so risk managers should be familiar with the basic techniques of encryption.

Role of risk manager in record keeping

A risk manager must learn to control and assess the documentation process in order to minimize liability exposures in this area. There are a number of basic strategies for doing so. To begin with, the risk manager will often review the incident history in the hopes of identifying trends. The style and format of the organization's records should be subject to regular review, and the risk manager should conduct a periodic review of all the organizational protocols related to documentation. The risk manager should also take a close look at the instances in the recent past in which the documentation of the organization has been problematic. The risk manager may want to review the notes from any meetings of the medical records committee in order to gain an understanding of the manner in which documentation problems have been handled in the past.

Basic steps of emergency management

The basic steps of emergency management are prevention, planning and preparation, implementation and response, and recovery. Prevention is essentially the creation of a culture that responds appropriately and effectively to emergencies. Part of prevention is the implementation of strong internal reporting systems so that information about risks can be made available to managers and executives. Planning and preparation entail the maintenance of a rapid response system for emergencies. Emergency response should be tested regularly. Every member of the emergency response team should understand his or her role and responsibilities. Implementation and response are the initiation of the emergency response plan as soon as possible. Part of response is having an effective public relations department. Finally, in the recovery phase, the institution becomes fully operational again as quickly as possible, a financial recovery is begun, and any injuries suffered by staff have been addressed.

Vulnerability to emergencies

Effect of design and location of healthcare facility
A risk manager needs to ensure that his or her facility has taken any necessary steps to mitigate risk related to the location or design of the business. For instance, buildings that are placed near fault lines should be examined for their susceptibility to earthquake. The seismic code (i.e., the requirements for buildings in earthquake-prone zones) was updated recently, and buildings that were erected prior to this update may be somewhat more vulnerable. It can be extremely expensive to retrofit a building to make it more resistant to earthquakes, however, so the risk manager will have to weigh the benefits of this process against the cost. One alternative to overhauling the design of the building is to create a cache of emergency supplies, like canned foods or medical equipment. If the facility is vulnerable to flooding, the risk manager should consider adding some structures to reduce the risks of damage, as for instance earth or concrete aqueducts or barriers.

Effective training
The risk manager is responsible for training staff to respond effectively to emergencies. Indeed, employees must understand both how to reduce their own risk of loss and how to reduce the risk of injury to patients. However, even though the staff members of the facility should be trained to act in response to a crisis, this does not necessarily mean that the staff will be in control in the event of an emergency. Instead, it is typically the local emergency planning council that assumes authority over the emergency response program. The risk manager and the other executives of the healthcare facility should cultivate relationships with the leaders of the local emergency planning council. Moreover, the risk manager should have contacts with all of the essential service providers (e.g., water, gas, electricity, phone). If appropriate, risk managers should emphasize to managers of these utility services that the facility has special needs and should receive priority in the event of an emergency.

Insurance coverage for protecting against loss during emergencies

In the event of an emergency, one of the chief responsibilities of the risk manager is to limit the amount of financial damage. One way to do this ahead of time is to review the insurance held by the institution and identify any gaps in coverage. For instance, the property and business interruption insurance held by medical facilities is usually quite inclusive, but some policies do contain exclusions that can reduce coverage after an emergency. The risk manager may also want to review the directors' and officers' liability; general, professional, and auto liability; workers' compensation; and aviation policies. When gaps are discovered in the facility's coverage, the risk manager should discuss with senior management whether it makes sense to eliminate them. In some cases, the risk of loss will not be worth the expense of increasing the coverage.

Emergency planning and preparation

The emergency plans drafted by a risk management department should be succinct and clear. The written versions of the plan should be reviewed by the major executives and the relevant department heads. Moreover, the plan should be drafted with input from the emergency department, medical staff, nursing staff, and security personnel. The risk manager may also want to order a hazard vulnerability analysis, which is a comprehensive assessment of the structural risks in a facility. There is a standard form for this analysis issued by the American Society for Healthcare Engineering (ASHE). This form asks the risk manager to consider the known risks, the risks that are evident from an evaluation of historical data, and the risks that are indicated by manufacturers or vendors. ASHE defines as a risk anything that creates the possibility of a threat to life and/or health, the possibility of damage or failure, the loss of community trust, disruption of services, financial impact, or legal issues. With respect to preparedness, the ASHE analysis asks the risk manager to consider the status of current plans, the training status, insurance, the availability of back-up systems, and community resources.

Integration of emergency response plans with community plans

According to Environment of Care Standard EC 4.10, organizations accredited by the Joint Commission must collaborate with community emergency planning and management agencies when composing and testing their own emergency response plans. Meeting this responsibility, as well as the strictures of the Centers for Medicare and Medicaid Services, is most easily accomplished by participation in a local emergency planning council. The general list of community groups with whom the facility should have contact includes emergency medical services, utilities, suppliers, contractors, and public safety agencies. One of the most important community liaisons for healthcare facilities is the Amateur Radio Emergency Services (ARES), which provides communication resources in times of need.

ICS

The incident command system (ICS), which is a standard procedure for emergency management, was developed by FIRESCOPE (Firefighting Resources of California Organized for Potential Emergencies) as a method of responding to wildfires. This program became the core of the Hospital Emergency Incident Command System (HEICS). The five major functions of the ICS command structure are command, operations, planning, logistics, and finance and administration. The command function is the locus of orders during the emergency. It is headed by the incident commander, who oversees the immediate response to problems. The planning function is the gathering of information related to the event. Planning also includes the initiation of support staff systems and the creation of a labor pool. The operations function is the set of activities concerned with directing emergency care, coordinating patient care, and facilitating evacuation procedures. The logistics function is the management of utility systems and supply distribution related to patient care. Logistics also includes food service and damage control. The finance and administration function is the tasks associated with funding immediate responses, recovery expenses, and overseeing claims management and liability control.

Emergency operations center

In the emergency operations center, the activities of the incident command system are coordinated and communicated. The selection of an appropriate site for the emergency operations center is an important decision. It should be close enough for communication to be easy, but far enough away that it is not likely to be affected by the emergency. In addition, there should be an alternate location in case the planned location cannot be used. Each emergency operations center should contain activity logs, communications equipment, essential references, and survival supplies. Moreover, staff should be trained in the basic procedures of the emergency operations center so that they will know what to expect in the event of an emergency.

Drills and practice events

Total preparation for emergencies must entail numerous drills and rehearsals so that every staff member knows his or her job and any unforeseen problems are identified and resolved. Any facility that is subsidized by the Joint Commission must have an emergency preparedness drill every four to eight months. In addition, the Joint Commission requires at least one drill every year. It is not necessary for every drill to fully simulate an emergency: many facilities conduct what are known as tabletop drills, in which staff members are given a written description of an urgent situation and asked to plan a response. It should be noted that drills and practice events cannot be totally successful unless the results are discussed and evaluated afterwards.

Implementation of emergency response systems

One of the key elements of an emergency response system is the designation of command. Usually, the emergency commander is the highest-ranking manager available, but the organization should have a clear plan for assigning authority, as well as a protocol for transferring authority when necessary. The implementation of the emergency response system should include a plan for internal communication; any stakeholders in the response should have a means of receiving updated information quickly. There should also be a clear protocol for communicating with external parties. For instance, there should be a designated spokesperson and location for briefings. The communications team should be able to draft and release information as soon as possible. Moreover, the communications team should be good at coordinating the efforts of government and nonprofit aid agencies.

Recovery process following an emergency

Much as a healthcare facility should develop a clear plan for responding to an emergency, it should also have a similar plan for recovering afterwards. There should be a clear plan for shutting down the incident command center, for instance, as well as collecting the records and data that will aid in future emergency response. The recovery team should be prepared to help employees deal with emotional or physical trauma, and should have a plan for reopening after repairs and renovations are complete. Indeed, the recovery team should be ready to call in building inspectors to confirm that the facility is ready for use. Finally, the recovery team should be prepared to communicate effectively and comprehensively with the media during the recovery process.

Donabedian's seven pillars of healthcare quality

The writer Avedis Donabedian outlined seven pillars of healthcare quality: efficacy, efficiency, optimality, acceptability, legitimacy, equity, and cost. Efficacy is the improvement of a patient's overall health. Efficiency is the achievement of the greatest results for the least expense. Optimality is striking the appropriate balance between costs and benefits. Acceptability is the capacity to make changes according to the patient's desires. Legitimacy is the provision of care that is positive for all people. Equity is the fair distribution of care. Finally, cost is the maximization of the cost-benefit ratio without sacrificing patient well-being in any way.

Benchmarking the total number of claims and potential claims

Every risk manager should benchmark the total number of claims and the total number of potential claims. The total number of claims is perhaps the best single performance indicator of the safety and risk program at an institution. Risk managers typically plot this information on a line graph, which can then be used to track the volume of claims against the institution. However, in many cases the total number of claims is so small that variations from month to month or even year to year are statistically insignificant. Moreover, it may be difficult to draw direct conclusions from the total number of claims because claims are a response to events that happened at some time in the past. In other words, a sudden increase in the number of claims may not be indicative of a greater amount of professional error or misconduct. Benchmarking the total number of potential claims, which is generally defined as the number of events after which the risk manager identifies the possibility of a claim or after which there is an identifiable harm to the patient, is often a better source of information. Keeping a count of the number of potential claims helps the organization decide the extent to which it should settle complaints before litigation ensues.

Benchmarking the costs of claims and risk

Every risk manager should benchmark the cost to the organization of claims and the total cost of risk. The total cost of claims should include expense and indemnity dollars paid and reserved. Indemnity costs generally include any funds required to settle with the plaintiff, as for instance pain and suffering, medical cost, and lost wages. The expense costs typically include any money spent on investigation, including attorneys' fees, expert witness fees, and the cost of depositions. Risk managers also keep track of the total cost of risk, which includes all operating units and lines of insurance coverage. Risk managers are often able to obtain more informative data by categorizing potential claims by event type or cause. However, the numbers of potential claims may already be small, and breaking it down into smaller groups may render the data meaningless.

PDCA cycle

The PDCA (plan, do, check, act) cycle is a method for refining processes to more nearly achieve a desired outcome. As the name suggests, the PDCA cycle has four basic steps: establishing goals and defining the changes necessary to achieve those goals, putting these changes into place, assessing the results of these changes, and solidifying the changes (i.e., renewing the PDCA cycle). Of course, the PDCA cycle requires accurate metrics. For most healthcare facilities, the recently introduced prospective patient safety measurements are an excellent tool. Whichever set of measurements is used, the facility must be sure that it is well-rounded so that a complete picture of the process is created.

Good catches and near misses

To improve the quality of the data related to sentinel events, many hospitals track events that do not result in loss, but which could or almost do. These are generally referred to as near misses and good catches. A near miss is defined by the Joint Commission as an event that did not have a significant outcome on this occasion, but which could if it happens in the future. A good catch, on the other hand, is an event that would have hurt the patient but which was halted before this could occur. Tracking near misses and good catches can tell the organization whether it has been unusually lucky or unlucky with regard to actual sentinel events, and can also indicate some areas in which the organization will need to improve its performance. This sort of tracking can be especially useful for small institutions which may not have enough claims to make the data statistically significant.

Risk management

In healthcare, risk management relates to all of the various risks incurred by the organization. It is important for the risk management program to include a well-defined set of policies and procedures, and for the program to have sufficient scope to cover all the potential risks. The discipline of risk management has only developed over the past half-century. In large part, it was spurred by an epidemic of malpractice cases in the 1970s. In 1980, the American Society for Healthcare Risk Management was established to promote sound strategies for protection against accidental loss. These strategies have coalesced into a general program known as enterprise risk management, which includes coverage for political, legal, regulatory, and financial risk. Another major catalyst in the development of healthcare risk management programs was the publication in 1999 of *To Err is Human: Building a Safer Health System*, an exposition of a study conducted by the Institute of Medicine. This study suggested that medical errors were both more prevalent and more costly than had previously been thought.

Risk management program

To be effective, a risk management program must include certain structural elements. For instance, every risk management program must include a comprehensive set of policies and procedures so that it will be applied consistently throughout the organization. Moreover, there must be an organized system for communicating the activities of the program to any interested parties. A risk management program should have a well-defined scope, and should include specific strategies for handling the risks associated with patients, employees, regulatory agencies, property, and vehicles. Finally, an effective risk management program will have a clear chain of authority so that there is no confusion as to the duties of various officers or the seat of responsibility.

<u>Authority</u>
In order for a risk management program to be effective, the head of the program must have enough authority to make any necessary changes in policy or procedure. Moreover, the risk

manager must be given access to whatever information will help him or her in this work, and at times this information may be sensitive or confidential. The risk manager, then, will perforce be high in the organizational hierarchy. In most healthcare institutions, the risk manager will report directly either to the chief executive officer or to another very high-ranking official. If the highest-ranking risk manager is not at least as elevated on the organizational chart as a department manager, it may be difficult for the risk manager to exercise the necessary amount of influence to perform his or her job well. The tasks of risk management are divided among several departments: for instance, the workers compensation program might be administered by the human resource department, while insurance issues may be handled by the finance department. This model may be successful as long as each respective component of the risk management program has sufficient authority and scope to complete its mission.

Visibility

Risk managers often emphasize the "visibility" of an effective program, by which they mean the degree of recognition given to the program by the other employees of the healthcare institution. It is especially important for a risk management program to be highly visible within the organization so that employees at all levels will be aware of the best practices. Risk management requires the participation of every member of the organization, and therefore the effective risk manager must be good at promoting his or her efforts. There are some common strategies for promoting the work of the risk management department: for instance, risk management professionals may conduct workshops and other educational events, and may occupy reserved places on relevant organizational committees.

Communication

Communication has become even more important for risk management programs over the past couple of decades as healthcare institutions have become increasingly complex combinations of clinics, managed care facilities, physician practices, etc. These networks, commonly known as integrated delivery systems, have produced unexpected and unprecedented problems related to loss control, potential liability, and the management of insurance claims. For this reason, it has become increasingly important for risk managers to be an integral part of the mergers and acquisitions process. Some of these new conglomerations will be attended by new risks, and therefore should be supervised by a risk management professional. A risk manager is more likely than an executive to recognize possible risks and required insurance coverages.

Leadership positions

Chief executive officer: To be effective, a risk management program must be comprehensively integrated with the other departments of the healthcare organization. The responsibility for this integration lies with several of the top officials, each of whom has a slightly different role in the process. The chief executive officer (CEO) is a vital source of information and authority for the risk management program. In order to undertake many of his or her initiatives, the risk manager will require the support of the CEO. Moreover, the CEO will be intimately involved in any mergers and acquisitions made by the institution, and should therefore be in close contact with the risk manager.

Chief financial officer and quality management director: The chief financial officer (CFO) is instrumental in allocating funds for and managing the budget of the risk management department. For instance, the CFO will be responsible for soliciting and monitoring actuarial analyses and setting limits for self-insured retentions. Finally, the quality management director (also known as the performance improvement director) is charged with keeping the risk manager informed about any relevant events within the institution. Although the Joint Commission has asserted that the performance improvement and risk management departments should be separate, the heads of these departments must be in close consultation during the creation of patient safety initiatives and the performance of root cause analyses following sentinel events.

Patient safety director, compliance officer, infection control practitioner, and safety officer: The patient safety director of a healthcare organization may actually be a part of the risk management department. Regardless of his or her direct superior, he or she will be essential in the development of strategies to prevent loss and manage clinical risk. The compliance officer is in charge of ensuring that the facility obeys the Sarbanes-Oxley Act and the Health Insurance Portability and Accountability Act (HIPAA), and avoids Medicare abuse and fraud. This typically entails organizing workshops and other staff education initiatives. The infection control practitioner is responsible for providing information about infections, which are common sources of liability claims. The risk manager will often work in close consultation with the infection control practitioner to reduce the frequency of infections within the facility. Also, the infection control practitioner will be instrumental in creating processes to handle communicable diseases in the facility. Finally, the safety officer will coordinate with the risk manager on such issues as fire safety, management of hazardous materials, and emergency protocols. All of these activities must be performed in accordance with the standards of the Joint Commission. Risk managers will often require information from the institution's safety committee, which is typically headed by the safety officer.

Patient representative and personnel director: The patient representative, often referred to as the ombudsman, serves as a liaison between patients and the various departments of the healthcare facility. It is important for the risk manager to maintain a good relationship with the patient representative so that any recurrent complaints are considered in the development of risk management policies. The personnel director, otherwise known as the employee health nurse, is responsible for handling the workers compensation program, a task which includes keeping the risk manager informed about injuries and claims. Injury management programs are often a collaboration between the risk manager and personnel director.

Health information manager and medical director: The health information manager is the contact person for attorneys representing patients, and therefore can alert the risk manager about impending legal proceedings. In addition, the health information manager (also known as the medical records director) is responsible for developing the institution's protocols for maintaining and releasing documents, both of which are subjects of great interest to the risk manager. Finally, the medical director coordinates the efforts of the medical staff and the risk management department. This means that the medical director will be responsible for informing doctors and medical staff about risk management protocols and ensuring compliance. The medical director will also be charged with ensuring that the medical departments hire and transfer employees in accordance with sound risk management practices.

Patient accounts representative, nursing and departmental manager, and human resource director: The patient accounts representative is responsible for handling patient complaints related to billings and collection. Because these complaints are often rooted in complaints about care, they are often of interest to the risk manager. It is not uncommon for a complaint that begins with billing and collections to blossom into a liability issue for the medical staff. The nursing and departmental managers are essential resources of technical information for the risk manager. In addition, these managers are responsible for keeping their subordinates informed about risk management efforts. Finally, the human resource director is responsible for hiring in a manner that conforms to risk management protocols. This entails conducting comprehensive background checks and competency testing before hiring, as well as performance appraisals for current employees. The human resource director will also be an important contact for the risk manager on any liability claims related to discrimination, wrongful termination, or sexual harassment.

Accountability
The risk manager must be held accountable for the success of his or her program. Accountability is the necessary consequence of authority. There should be a list of the specific duties and responsibilities of the risk manager so that his or her performance can be assessed. Furthermore, the risk management program should have measurable goals so that its success or failure can be judged. In most organizations, the risk manager is subject to annual performance appraisals. It is also common for the risk manager to submit an annual report to the organization's senior management. In this report, the risk manager will lay out the major initiatives of the risk management program over the past year, as well as the most important recent events.

Addressing risks
Patient care-related risks: A comprehensive risk management program will address risks related to patients, medical staff, other employees, property, and finances. For most organizations, the majority of claims will have to do with patient care. This trend has been particularly evident in the past decade, as both the number of claims and the average settlement per claim have risen. A risk management program must be adept at gathering information, managing loss, financing medical professional liability risk, and handling claims. The majority of claims stemming from patient care will be related to improper medical treatment, but the risk manager will also need to know how to deal with claims related to confidentiality and the release of patient medical information. The risk manager should also be aware of the potential for abuse and neglect of patients by other patients, staff, or visitors to the facility. This category also includes the theft of patient valuables, patient participation in research studies, and patient discharges and referrals for necessary services by third parties.

Medical staff-related risks: Many of the risks that fall under the purview of a risk management program are related to the medical staff. Indeed, the most serious risks are almost always to do with doctors and other medical practitioners. The risk manager should be intimately involved in the hiring, appointment, and promotion of medical staff. To this end, the risk manager should be a part of the peer review and performance enhancement programs for medical staff. The risk management program will need to have a comprehensive and explicit program for investigating and disciplining medical staff. In particular, the risk management program will need to have a strong and clear system for identifying impaired practitioners. Finally, the risk manager should be conversant with how different managed care plans handle physician gatekeeper obligations and incentives.

Employee-related risks: In the context of a healthcare facility, employee-related risks are defined as those pertaining to personnel besides doctors and medical staff. The risk manager must be concerned with maintaining a safe work environment so as to diminish instances of occupational illness and injury. When injuries and illnesses do occur, however, the risk management program must include a comprehensive and equitable workers compensation program. To this, the risk manager must stay abreast of the workers compensation rules and regulations of the federal Occupational Safety and Health Administration and the state alike. In addition, the risk manager will have to deal with problems related to discrimination in hiring and promotion and complaints filed with the Equal Employment Opportunity Commission. In these areas, the risk manager will be particularly reliant on the assistance of the human resource department.

Property-related risks: Often, it is assumed that risk management has only to do with adverse events affecting patients or staff. The maintenance and protection of the healthcare institution's property is also within the purview of the risk manager, however. A healthcare institution may have extremely valuable physical property, both in the form of buildings and equipment. The risk manager must establish insurance policies to protect property from damage or loss caused by fire, flood, or other natural disaster. There will need to be separate insurance policies for the valuable data resources of the institution, as well. A healthcare institution cannot afford to have its operations delayed by problems with data retrieval or storage. Another property-related risk that must be considered by the risk manager is the possibility of loss or theft of cash and valuable possessions belonging to patients. The risk management department must establish a specific protocol for handling allegations and investigations of theft.

Financial risks: A few of the financial risks of a healthcare institution are placed under the responsibility of the risk management department. To begin with, the risk manager is in charge of handling any liability of the board of directors or officers that is imposed by claims made by shareholders or others. The fulfillment of this responsibility will require the risk manager to be conversant with the corporate structure of the institution, as well as the relevant local, state, and federal laws. Another financial risk that is the responsibility of the risk management department is the risk inherent in complex managed care organizations. These financial risks may be defined as aggregate if the total cost of providing medical services is higher than expected, or may be specific if the cost of providing services to a single subscriber is considerably higher than expected. There are numerous strategies for transferring and distributing this risk.

Miscellaneous risks: There are a few other minor sources of risk that are typically considered the responsibility of the risk management department. For instance, the risk management department may be charged with protecting the vehicles used by the facility, which may include ambulances, cars, trucks, vans, and even helicopters or airplanes. Many large healthcare institutions also deem it necessary to obtain insurance coverage against loss or damage caused by terrorism. At the very least, organizations that are considered vulnerable should create elaborate disaster and emergency preparation plans in order to guard against the possibility of an attack. A final area of concern for risk managers is the management of hazardous materials. The organization must have specific protocols for the handling, storage, and disposal of toxic and radioactive materials.

Department budgets
Depending on the size of the institution, a risk manager may be responsible for generating and adhering to a specific budget for his or her department. When drafting a budget, the risk manager needs to consider the size and significance of the facility's greatest liabilities.

Obviously, the previous budgets will be the most important source of information on this subject. When these records are not available, or when changes within the institution have rendered them obsolete, the risk manager may be able to obtain useful information from competing institutions. Much of this data is in the public domain. The risk manager may also look at the budgets of other departments within the same institution to develop a sense of the appropriate scale for his or her own budget.

Steps of risk management process

The process of risk management may be simplified into five steps: identify and analyze loss exposures; weigh alternative risk techniques; choose the best technique or techniques; implement and assess and improve the implemented program. During the identification of loss exposures, the risk manager will have to consider the types of exposures, as well as the appropriate methods for identifying these. Once the exposures have been identified, the risk manager will need to determine the significance of the risk and the extent to which it affects the organizational objectives. The manager will then need to decide whether it is more appropriate to control the risk or to finance it after it happens. The risk manager will then select the optimal strategy according to a specific and unique set of selection criteria. Finally, after the program has been implemented, the manager will need to monitor it according to the most appropriate criteria.

Identification and analysis of loss exposures

The first step in the process of risk management is the identification and analysis of loss exposures. The losses to which a healthcare facility is exposed are manifold: financial, capital, and intangible losses may all occur. The primary method of identifying risk is a sound incident reporting system, in which employees alert the risk management department about any practices or protocols that may be creating risk. Some healthcare institutions have elaborate electronic incident reporting systems, while others rely on simple paper records. A healthcare institution may also receive valuable alerts from patient complaints or from the results of patient surveys. Similarly, a facility may obtain information from generic occurrence screening, in which a team of experts review completed cases to determine whether care has been optimal. Other sources of information that may be valuable during the identification and analysis of loss exposures are prior claims data; state licensure surveys; contracts; Joint Commission surveys; and discussions with staff, managers, and employees.

Weighing alternative risk techniques

After loss exposures have been identified and analyzed, the risk manager will begin to weigh the possible strategies for mitigating these risks. These strategies fall into two categories: risk control and risk financing. Risk control strategies attempt to prevent or minimize the damage caused by losses, while risk financing strategies accept the inevitability of loss and concentrate on efforts to pay for them. The major risk control techniques are non-insurance transfer, segregation of loss exposures, loss reduction, loss prevention, and exposure avoidance. Risk financing typically involves either risk retention or risk transfer. The choice of strategy will depend in part on the extent to which the risk manager believes that he or she can prevent the loss, and the moral and financial consequences of allowing a loss to happen. For instance, losses that entail injury, illness, or death cannot be tolerated at all, and must be prevented as much as possible. On the other hand, a risk manager would probably be willing to accept some loss of property due to theft or user error, and would decline to endorse excessively expensive prevention plans and insurance.

Risk control techniques

<u>Exposure avoidance, loss prevention, and loss reduction</u>
In the risk control technique called exposure avoidance, the risk manager attempts to prevent the risk from occurring at all. Of course, this strategy is only viable when the loss can realistically be prevented. One way to avoid a risk is simply to stop providing the service that creates it. For instance, if a healthcare facility wants to avoid losses related to blood transfusions, it could just stop performing this operation. Obviously, this strategy cannot be applied to every risk, or the facility would lose its reason for being. Loss prevention, by contrast, is an attempt to reduce the frequency of the loss. Loss prevention is fundamental to risk management, and typically includes changes to policies and procedures. Loss reduction is an attempt to reduce the severity rather than the frequency of loss. One of the best methods of loss reduction is good communication, because this allows errors and accidents to be identified and handled as soon as possible. Loss reduction is also aided by prompt investigation and response to incidents.

<u>Segregation of loss exposures and non-insurance transfer</u>
One of the less common techniques for risk control is loss exposure, in which the activities of the organization are compartmentalized so that an error occurring in one area will not affect others. In order for this strategy to be effective, each activity must be performed in multiple departments of the facility so that an error in one area will not prevent the same service from being performed elsewhere. For instance, a healthcare facility will often maintain copies of electronic records in several locations. Another technique for risk control is non-insurance transfer, in which the risk manager uses contracts, leases, and other agreements to divest the institution of legal responsibility for risk. The use of this technique can be problematic, however, as the courts have sometimes declined to enforce transfers that are against public policy or are deemed unfair to the transferee.

Selecting a risk management technique

To select the proper risk management technique, one must attempt to predict the consequences of each viable option. In addition, one must consider these consequences in the light of the organization's specific objectives. The extent to which each option contributes to the objectives of the organization must be balanced with its cost; no institution can afford an ideal risk management program. In most cases, the risk management department will opt for an array of techniques, including risk control and risk financing. It is common for a healthcare institution to obtain a small amount of insurance to cover patient care liability risk, and to focus the rest of its efforts on preventing loss and reducing the impact of those losses that do occur. The long-term goal of the risk management department is to diminish the amount of loss but to maintain a realistic view of the amount of loss likely to occur.

Implementing risk management techniques

After the optimal battery of risk management techniques has been selected, the next step is to implement the program. This step is the first to require a great deal of participation from other departments within the organization. The risk management department may make recommendations and even demands of the other departments, but it will be up to the managers of those diverse departments to implement the strategies. During this process, the risk management department should collaborate and advise the other departments as much as possible. For instance, the risk management department is often a good source of information about various insurers, as well as the proper limits for deductibles and coverage.

Risk financing strategies

Risk financing strategies accept the inevitability of loss and concentrate on paying for it. It may be defined as risk retention or risk transfer. In risk retention, the healthcare institution generates funds to pay for loss. This strategy is often used when the risk cannot be avoided, minimized, or transferred. It is also useful for dealing with relatively insignificant losses, and especially for losses that are easy to predict and quantify. Loss retention may entail setting aside a particular sum of money at regular intervals, securing insurance, or borrowing money to prepare for possible losses. Risk transfer, on the other hand, involves placing the financial responsibility for loss with another entity, as for instance an insurance company. Of course, risk transfer does not entail the transfer of legal responsibility for accidents. It is common for hospitals to acquire medical professional liability insurance against malpractice suits, though the legal responsibility for negligence or error remains with the institution.

Monitoring and improving risk management programs

The final steps in any risk management program are to monitor and improve the strategies after they have been implemented. This is a cooperative process involving risk managers, executives, medical staff, and department heads. The evaluation of the risk management program should involve a diverse array of assessment tools so that the full range of effects can be observed. The focus of assessment should always be to find ways in which the program can improve. The performance of the program should be measured against specific benchmarks, and these benchmarks should be established before the initiation of the program. A risk management program may make use of internal or external benchmarks, i.e., comparisons with other departments in the same institution or with similar departments in other institutions. Claims data is often a good source of information for the purposes of benchmarking.

Identifying areas that require assessment

In order to expedite the assessment of a risk management program, the most vital areas should be considered first. In other words, the risk manager should examine those areas that attract the most attention and have the potential for the most loss. There should also be assessments for the entire organization, as well as for individual departments and specific functions within those departments. Moreover, there should be assessments for each of the various aspects of the program, including the financial, clinical, and operational. The risk manager will be alert to the ways in which assessment suggests the need for specialization in different departments.

Analysis of current risk management systems

The risk manager will need to take an honest look at the institution's current risk management systems before he or she can make recommendations for improvement. The risk manager will need to make a comprehensive map of the personnel and their responsibilities, as well as the relationships between the various departments. The risk manager will also need to create inventories of the educational credentials of key employees, the operational relationships between employees, the scope of services provided by each department, and the presence of consultants or other external collaborators. The risk manager should also inventory the relevant information technology programs, the human resources protocols, and the degree to which all of these systems are applied consistently throughout the facility. Finally, the risk manager should catalog all of the loss runs, loss assessment data, and the records of regulatory agency inspections.

Assessing compliance with current risk management program

As part of the initial assessment of current risk management systems, the risk manager will need to evaluate the extent to which the systems are in compliance with regulatory agencies and the managed care market. For instance, it may be necessary for the employees of a healthcare facility to maintain particular certifications, or to attend regular training sessions. Moreover, the risk management department may be required to submit periodic reports to regulatory bodies or insurance providers. This exercise is important not only because it indicates areas that need improvement, but because it reminds the risk management team of the rules that must be followed during the subsequent program development. The risk manager may also use the compliance requirements to develop useful metrics. In general, the risk manager should attend to the ease with which the organization is able to respond and comply with external mandates.

The assessments of the current risk management program should include measures of the frequency, severity, and overall consequences of each incident. An ideal assessment will also include a summary of the areas in which the program can improve, and the best practices for each relevant task. With regard to each of the organization's tasks, the risk manager should consider both how well the task is performed and how well the performance is documented. The risk management program should strive for both excellent performance and comprehensive record-keeping. After a sufficient amount of assessment, the risk manager will begin to lead the implementation of the program. He or she should decide the order in which program elements are to be implemented. It is not always appropriate to initiate the most important elements first. For instance, incident reporting systems may represent only a small part of the overall program, but must be up and running before the success of the other program elements may be evaluated.

Composing a risk management program plan

One of the most important steps in the formation of a risk management program is the composition of the program plan. The program plan should include a summary of the intentions, structure, and techniques. The general goals of the program should be supported by specific objectives: measurable performance targets that must be met in order for the general goals to be achieved. The program plan should emphasize consistency of purpose throughout the organization so that all departments are pulling in the same direction. The program plan should also include descriptions of how information will move through the system: that is, how directives will proceed out from the risk management department to other areas of the organization, and how alerts, complaints, and incident reports will be transmitted back to the risk management department.

Building support for a risk management program

The success of a risk management program requires buy-in from every member of the organization, not just the members of the risk management department. A high level of participation requires excellent communication between the risk management department and the other employees. In addition, the risk management program needs to have credibility with the rest of the organization. This credibility is earned by leading staff members in training and orientation sessions, and by remaining accessible to the rest of the organization. In general, it is best for the risk management department to emphasize loss prevention, as this technique is generally the easiest for other employees to understand and apply. The risk management department can also build rapport with the rest of the organization by contributing to compliance with state licensing departments and the Joint Commission's National Patient Safety Goals.

Risk manager's responsibilities

The particular tasks of a risk manager will depend in large part on the size and structure of the organization, as well as the preferred methods of risk management. In large organizations, the head of the department may be known as the chief risk officer, and may be responsible for financial planning as well as risk management. In other organizations, the risk manager will be known as a patient safety officer, and will focus on handling patient complaints and improving service provision. As risk management has become a more established field, there has been an effort to codify the knowledge base and required tasks for the profession. Most notably, the American Society for Healthcare Risk Management (ASHRM) used the results of an industry-wide survey to divide the responsibilities of the risk manager into six categories: loss prevention and reduction, claims management, risk financing, regulatory and accreditation compliance, risk management operations, and bioethics.

Risk manager's roles

Loss prevention and reduction
The greatest responsibility for a risk manager is usually loss prevention and reduction. For instance, a risk manager may be responsible for developing risk identification systems, like medical record reviews, protocols for handling complaints, and incident reporting systems. The risk manager may also be responsible for coordinating the loss prevention and reduction efforts of multiple departments. Loss prevention and reduction may entail the composition of statistical and qualitative reports, root cause analysis, and failure mode and effects analysis. The risk manager will often be responsible for developing training programs for staff, as well as for investigating and responding to claims made by staff members. Finally, the risk management department may be responsible for developing the organizational protocols related to informed consent, confidentiality, and the response to sentinel events.

Claims management

The risk management department is usually responsible for handling possible or actual claims, whether during the investigation or the resolution phase. The risk manager will be responsible for alerting the insurance carrier to impending claims, as well as handling all the related paperwork. If an investigation of the claim is required, it may be led by the risk management department. The risk manager should be available to coordinate the response to requests for information and employee interviews during the investigation. The risk manager may be required to oversee the activities of the defense counsel or third-party administrators. The risk manager may need to establish expense and indemnity reserves, and may be responsible for approving settlements. Finally, it is often the job of the risk manager to act as a liaison between the senior management and the department affected by the claim.

Risk financing

Risk managers are often responsible for handling the financing of losses, both by determining the amount of money required and the method of payment. For instance, the risk manager may be required to maintain the organization's batch of exposure data, and may be charged with handling the applications for insurance coverage. This may entail working with underwriters, actuaries, and insurance brokers. During this process, the risk manager will be instrumental in determining the appropriate coverage limits, deductibles, and forms of coverage. The risk manager must be familiar with the various forms of risk financing, including commercial insurance, retention, and captive insurance. Finally, once a risk financing program has been implemented, the risk manager is usually in charge of monitoring and improving it.

Regulatory and accreditation compliance

A risk manager is responsible for many of the tasks involved in regulatory and accreditation compliance. He or she must be familiar with the Americans with Disabilities Act, the Safe Medical Devices Act, the Emergency Medical Treatment and Labor Act, the Health Care Quality Improvement Act, the Health Insurance Portability and Accountability Act, and the Patient Self-Determination Act. In addition, the risk manager will need to be familiar with the regulations advanced by the Institute of Medicine, the Occupational Safety and Health Administration, and the Joint Commission. In particular, the risk manager must attend to the Joint Commission's strictures regarding sentinel events and national patient safety standards. Finally, the risk manager will be tasked with ensuring compliance with applicable rules related to the reporting of deaths.

Risk management operations and bioethics

Much of the work of a risk manager is related to running his or her department. For instance, a risk manager will be responsible for developing the organizational risk management plan and a set of approved policies. The risk manager will also be responsible for hiring, training, and supervising the risk management staff. The risk manager usually heads the risk management and patient safety committees in large institutions, and must both establish departmental goals and chart the progress towards these goals. The risk manager also has a number of responsibilities that fall under the heading of bioethics. These include responsibilities related to the withdrawal of life support, research on human subjects, brain death, advance directives, and do-not-resuscitate orders. In addition, the risk management department may be asked to handle unforeseen ethical dilemmas that arise within the organization.

Risk manager's roles in various settings

Acute care hospital
The specific role and responsibilities of a risk manager are largely dependent on the institution in which he or she is working. The largest portion of risk managers are employed by acute care hospitals. An acute care hospital typically has anywhere from 100 to 500 beds. Acute care hospitals are subdivided into teaching hospitals, large facilities with several residency programs, and community hospitals which are smaller and may not have any residency programs at all. In very large acute care facilities, the risk manager is usually tasked with a limited number of related areas, as for instance infection control and patient safety. If the facility is small, the risk manager may also be placed in charge of corporate compliance. Small acute-care facilities usually have commercial insurance, which drastically reduces the amount of paperwork that must be completed by the risk management department. With regard to risk financing, the manager at a small acute care facility may only need to organize exposure data and to handle applications and renewals.

Academic medical center
The role of a risk manager at an academic medical center is somewhat unique. These institutions are often engaged in research, which introduces a number of specific risk exposures. It is common for the risk management department to have separate leaders for the academic and the medical branches of the facility. The risk exposures of an academic facility are further multiplied by the relatively high number of practitioners involved in patient care. At an academic medical center, a patient may be treated by students, specialists, residents, and others. The amount of turnover at an academic medical center is likely to be high, which can create problems for the risk manager. In addition, the frequent changes in staff make the education and training aspects of risk management especially important. Unlike in acute care medical centers, the claims management in an academic institution is generally handled by the risk management department. Finally, the compliance and accreditation issues faced by an academic medical center are often very complex, and may therefore be handled by a specialist.

Integrated delivery system
An integrated delivery system may include group practices, specialty clinics, acute care facilities, and home care services. These complex organizations may range over wide geographic areas and have ornate corporate structures. Obviously, then, the work of a risk manager for an integrated delivery system will be highly variable. In a typical arrangement, a corporate risk manager leads the department, with several middle managers in charge of claims management, risk prevention and reduction, and compliance. Integrated delivery systems are run as large businesses, and are therefore more likely to be involved in mergers and acquisitions. For this reason, the risk manager of such a facility will need to be very familiar with contracts and risk financing.

Multi-facility healthcare system
A multi-facility healthcare system is one in which a single organization is in charge of several different facilities, each of which provides roughly the same services. The risk manager may have to deal with diverse institutions, which may have distinct cultures and loss exposures due to their locations, patient demographics, and staff. Moreover, risk management may be carried out on an operational level by managers at each facility, with general direction from a corporate risk manager. This corporate risk manager is also likely to be responsible for the risk financing activities, though claims activity is usually handled

by specialist staff. The activities related to bioethics and compliance are generally handled at each facility, with the corporate risk manager acting as a consultant and liaison between the facility managers.

Ambulatory care organization
Public health facilities, specialty clinics, self-contained surgical centers, walk-in medical clinics, and even physician practices all may be defined as ambulatory care organizations. Obviously, then, the structure and duties of the risk management department may be highly variable. One risk that is unique to this sort of facility is that of poor post-treatment care. The patients of an ambulatory care center will be returning home after treatment, so the facility must have a comprehensive and well-enforced set of protocols related to following up. Another unique feature of the ambulatory care facility is a lack of advanced infection control, biomedical, and safety equipment, which can create risk. Ambulatory care organizations are likely to see a broad spectrum of patients, and therefore should have an excellent program for receiving and responding to patient questions and complaints. Finally, in most ambulatory care organizations, the responsibilities related to accreditation and compliance are not assigned to the risk manager.

Physician practice or group
The primary responsibilities of a risk manager for a physician practice or group are loss prevention, patient safety, risk financing, and claims management. Physician practices are subject to risks associated with patient privacy, confidentiality of records, and unexpected patient responses. A physician practice is likely to be a smaller enterprise, and so the work of the risk manager there is usually less specialized. The risk manager may be tasked with establishing procedural standards, and is likely to work on the premises of the practice. The risk manager is likely to be the contact person for patients who have complaints, and may be integral to the process of investigating and settling claims.

Long-term care facility
The role and responsibilities of a risk manager in a long-term care facility vary widely depending on the complexity of the organization. Long-term care facilities are sometimes located within acute care facilities, but they may also be in separate buildings. The risks associated with long-term care facilities are unique because of how long patients tend to stay in these facilities. Also, the amount of care provided to the patients in these facilities tends to vary widely, so it is very important for the risk manager to ensure that all employees are working within their scope of practice. Long-term care facilities are more likely to be subject to allegations of negligence, so the risk manager should be particularly conscious of avoiding this sort of liability.

Education requirements for healthcare risk managers

Although there are not yet many risk management programs offered by universities, most risk managers have achieved at least a bachelor's degree in a related field, and half of these go on to earn a master's degree, as well. Moreover, a risk manager must constantly be seeking to continue his or her education. The most common way is through programs offered by the American Society for Healthcare Risk Management (ASHRM), which are available to members as well as non-members. The most basic certification offered by the ASHRM is the Barton Certificate of Healthcare Risk Management, which is composed of three modules covering the basic elements of the profession. For professionals who desire even more instruction, the ASHRM offers advanced seminars on regulatory changes and risk financing topics throughout the year. Many of the larger healthcare liability insurance carriers also provide educational opportunities for their clients, and risk managers may participate in these.

Certification and licensure requirements for healthcare risk managers

At present, the only certification program for healthcare risk managers is the Certified Professional in Healthcare Risk Management (CPHRM) designation, which is administered by the American Hospital Association Certification Center and the American Society for Healthcare Risk Management (ASHRM). To achieve this qualification, a candidate must meet the education and work experience criteria, and must pass an examination. Outstanding achievement in the profession may be rewarded by the ASHRM with a designation as a Fellow, while especially high achievement may earn a designation as a Distinguished Fellow. A similar program is offered by the Insurance Institute of America, after completion of which a candidate may be awarded the Associate in Risk Management designation. To achieve this designation, however, the risk manager must pass examinations in risk assessment, risk control, and risk financing.

Claims and Litigation

Coverage determination

Before the claims process can begin in earnest, there must be a coverage determination. In other words, someone needs to decide whether the incident is covered by insurance. This is performed by the insurance company when the facility has commercial coverage, and by an appropriate external party when the facility is self-insured. To begin with, the evaluator will decide whether the person or people involved in the proposed claim are covered by insurance. The evaluator will then determine whether the loss occurred during the policy period. If so, he or she will judge whether the loss occurred in a covered location, and whether it is subject to any exclusions. The evaluator must then make sure that the types and amounts of damages are covered, and that the cause of the loss is covered as well. Finally, the evaluator will need to determine whether there are any other insurance policies that could cover the loss.

Responsibilities of risk manager and claims adjuster

The risk manager of a healthcare facility is responsible for monitoring the claims process, even those components which do not require his or her direct participation. There are five major elements of the claims process: reporting, investigation, management, and settlement or litigation. The responsibility for reporting the claim will be with the primary insurer if the facility holds a commercial insurance policy. Self-insured organizations will need to report claims themselves. The investigation process can contain many different steps, as for instance an initial assessment, an expert review, a medical record review, and a battery of interviews. Claims management typically entails a determination of liability and a decision as to whether the claim should be settled or defended. If the decision is to settle, the risk manager must ensure that appropriate documentation is collected. If the decision is to litigate, the risk manager will need to monitor the preparation for trial, including the creation of a public relations strategy and the preparation of witnesses. During the trial, the risk manager will need to be a liaison for the legal team.

Identifying and investigating claims

One of the fundamental elements of a risk management program is a set of procedures for identifying and investigating claims. The reporting of a claim begins when a member of the staff reports a possible claim to the risk management professional. Then, assuming the facility has commercial insurance, the risk manager will submit a report to the insurance carrier. At this point, the investigation of the claim will begin. If the risk manager is in charge of the investigation, he or she should conduct it while in consultation with a legal adviser. Not only will this ensure that the investigation stays on the right side of the law, but it will create attorney-client privilege protection for much of the investigation's contents. An investigation will usually begin with interviews of all the main parties to the event. The general rule is that any person who is in a position to provide relevant and material information should be interviewed.

Claims file management

Claims file management is an essential part of a risk manager's portfolio. When a claims audit occurs, it is crucial for the risk manager to have a strong file system. The standard file system is composed of the following categories: correspondence, investigation documentation, medical records, expert records, medical research, damages, legal papers, expenses, and reserve history. Each of these categories should be updated according to the same rules. Many risk managers find it useful to compose a cover sheet for each file, summarizing the most recent claim status, litigation, and indemnity and expense history. Within each claims file, there should be a loss reserve, or estimate of how much the claim will cost. Of course, it will also be necessary to pay the legal fees, conduct the investigation, and adjust the claim. In determining the amount of the loss reserve, a risk manager will typically take the following factors into account: demographics, the nature and extent of the injury, damages (i.e., total medical bills, possible future expenses), representation (i.e., whether the claimant has legal counsel), liability factors (i.e., ways in which the standard of care was not reached), and precedents (i.e., similar claims from the past).

Settlement or alternative dispute resolution

A risk manager must be fully aware of the various means of resolving claims. In some cases, the easiest way to resolve the claim is to pay a small amount of money, but the risk manager may want to avoid having the loss on the facility's permanent record. One way to avoid having the claim become a part of the legal record is to reach a settlement before trial. If the facility admits that it is liable for damages that resulted from a breach of the duty to maintain a standard of care, it is usually best to settle. The basic elements of a settlement are monetary compensation, additional treatment, and a release from future liability. In cases where liability is acknowledged but the amount of damages is in dispute, it may be necessary to use an alternative means of dispute resolution, as for instance mediation or arbitration. The alternative means of dispute resolution are distinguished by whether they are binding or nonbinding, i.e., whether the disputing parties are obliged to follow the direction of the third party.

Reporting insurance claims

Risk managers are required to report claims to several bodies. To begin with, any organization or insurance company that makes payment on behalf of a healthcare institution for injuries sustained by a patient during the course of medical treatment must report the details of the transaction to the National Practitioner Data Bank. In addition, these payments must be reported to the appropriate state licensing agency within a month of the payment. It is possible for patients to file claims against physicians through a state nursing or medical board. When such claims are made, the nursing or medical board will investigate the allegations according to the peer review process. As for risk managers, they are also responsible for reporting any claims to the peer review and quality improvement committees of their institution.

Claims-made and occurrence policies

Healthcare insurance policies may be written on a claims-made or an occurrence basis. The most common types of claims to be written on the claims-made basis are managed care errors and omissions and directors' and officers' liability. The most common types of claims to be written on an occurrence basis are automobile, property, and workers' compensation. On a claims-made form, the interval between the retroactive date and the commencement date of the current policy period is called the nose. The tail, also referred to as the extended reporting period, is an interval after the termination of the policy during which it is still active. The policy holder typically must pay extra for an extended reporting period to be added to the policy.

Chain of custody for potential evidence

In order for healthcare employees to maintain the ability to testify accurately and confidently about the evidence related to individual liability claims, an adequate chain of custody procedure must be in place at the facility. There are no specific requirements for the chain of custody in a healthcare facility or laboratory, but certain guidelines must be followed. To begin with, the chain of custody must be recorded by the facility at which the evidence originated, and this report should be comprehensive up until the responsibility for the evidence is transferred to another body. The chain of custody report should include the name and signature of each person who has removed the evidence from its place in storage. The report should also include the time, date, and reason for the removal.

Practice Test

Practice Questions

1. What are the four components of the SBAR situational briefing model?
    a. Situation, background, assessment, and recommendation
    b. Status, briefing, analysis, and reconnaissance
    c. Safety, bearing, argument, and rationale
    d. Scenario, basis, acquisition, and response

2. Which of the following is NOT one of the patient rights enumerated in the Patient Self-Determination Act?
    a. Patients have the right to refuse medical treatment.
    b. Patients have the right to facilitate decisions related to their own health care.
    c. Patients have the right to select their medication.
    d. Patients have the right to make advance health care directives.

3. What is one advantage of a voluntary error reporting system over a mandatory error reporting system?
    a. Mandatory systems are only targeted at very narrow areas of practice.
    b. Voluntary systems eliminate the need for communication among health care organizations.
    c. Voluntary systems elicit more reports from frontline practitioners.
    d. Mandatory systems discourage the reporting of nonfatal errors.

4. What, in particular, is the process chain in a laboratory subject to?
    a. Variability
    b. Delay
    c. Disorganization
    d. Conflict

5. A root cause analysis of inpatient suicides would be most likely to discover problems with
    a. staffing levels.
    b. staff orientation.
    c. the physical environment.
    d. the availability of information.

6. Which of the following is NOT one of the types of quality problem identified by the Institute of Medicine's National Roundtable on Health Care Quality?
    a. Misuse
    b. Abuse
    c. Overuse
    d. Underuse

7. Which of the following conditions must be met for a patient to no longer be deserving of service under the Emergency Medical Treatment and Active Labor Act?
    a. The patient must have provided the contact information of a person who can care for him upon discharge.
    b. The patient must be able to feed himself without special equipment.
    c. The patient must be alert.
    d. The patient must be able to communicate without special equipment.

8. Which of the following groups is least likely to report errors?
    a. Primary care physicians
    b. Support staff
    c. Independent contractors
    d. Nurses

9. What do hospitals that implement computerized provider order entry (CPOE) almost always see a decline in?
    a. Medication errors
    b. Diagnostic errors
    c. Adverse events
    d. Latent errors

10. Whenever possible, medication orders should be by
    a. weight.
    b. volume.
    c. dose.
    d. strength.

11. When a hospital official notes that most errors are occurring at the "sharp end," what does he mean?
    a. They involve surgical tools or knives.
    b. They occur in clusters.
    c. They occur during the interactions between caregivers and patients.
    d. They are more likely to occur during busy periods.

12. When does research suggest that people make fewer errors?
    a. When they perform several tasks at once
    b. When they work creatively
    c. When they work individually
    d. When they work in a team

13. Which of the following groups may request information from the Health Care Integrity and Protection Data Bank?
    a. Professional societies with formal peer review
    b. Quality improvement organizations
    c. Plaintiffs' attorneys
    d. State agencies

14. Which of the following factors is NOT included in a calculation of risk priority number?
    a. Severity of possible adverse effects
    b. Effectiveness of controls
    c. Likelihood of an adverse effect
    d. Cost of controls

15. Which of the following would be defined as a *sentinel event* by the Joint Commission?
    a. Radiation therapy 10 percent above the planned dose
    b. Suicide more than four days after discharge from a continuous care setting
    c. Moderate neonatal jaundice
    d. Hemolytic transfusion reaction caused by blood group incompatibility

16. Before conducting a safety audit in an emergency department, what does an administrator need to obtain first?
    a. A list of the employees in that department
    b. A map of the department
    c. A written set of safety standards
    d. Statistics on adverse events

17. Because of a doctor's poor handwriting, a prescription must be reworked before it leaves the pharmacy. Which of the following is true?
    a. The doctor should be reprimanded.
    b. The pharmacy should incorporate bar coding.
    c. The prescription should not count toward the pharmacy's yield.
    d. The error should be reported to the FDA.

18. Which of the following groups reports information to the Health Care Integrity and Protection Data Bank?
    a. Federal agencies
    b. Peer-review organizations
    c. Hospitals
    d. Medical malpractice payers

19. In general, how many steps should a failure modes and effects analysis proceed in each direction?
    a. One
    b. Two
    c. Five
    d. Ten

20. Why does the Healthcare Quality Improvement Act provide confidentiality and legal immunity for health care peer-review processes?
    a. To prevent malpractice suits
    b.. To discourage complaints by patients
    c. To encourage participation by physicians
    d. To maintain a sterile work environment

21. What is the first and most important step in a disclosure conversation?
    a. Assessing the patient's mood
    b. Admitting error and apologizing
    c. Discussing the root cause analysis
    d. Compensating the patient

22. If an at-risk patient is left unattended and has an adverse response to medication, what is this known as?
    a. A sentinel event
    b. An initiator
    c. A latent outcome
    d. A slip

23. How would the frequency of errors in a particular process be best displayed?
    a. Matrix diagram
    b. Pareto chart
    c. Affinity diagram
    d. Histogram

24. It has been determined that a hospital's blood transfusions are 99.7 percent error free. Which function can be used to determine the number of blood transfusions that are likely to be performed before an error is made?
    a. Binomial distribution
    b. Poisson distribution
    c. Negative binomial distribution
    d. Multinomial distribution

25. A hospital uses the same labels for all of its prescriptions, but these labels do not fit on the smallest containers, so employees must cut and paste the labels in a special way in order to fill the prescriptions. What is this an example of?
    a. Overproduction
    b. Queuing
    c. Work-in-progress
    d. Extra processing

26. A behavioral health specialist notices a particularly high number of restraint deaths at a facility. An analysis of the root causes of these events is most likely to indicate problems with
    a. equipment.
    b. staff orientation and training.
    c. staffing levels.
    d. alarm systems.

27. Which of the following is responsible for the most privacy violations of the Health Insurance Portability and Accountability Act?
    a. Improper disposal of data
    b. Data disclosed without the authorization of the patient
    c. Loss of data
    d. Physical theft of data

28. As much as possible, medications should be standardized. However, when this is impossible, what is it important to do?
    a. Assume that side effects will occur
    b. Warn clinicians about the potential for overdose
    c. Only use them as a last resort
    d. Differentiate them clearly

29. Which of the following is NOT one of the typical questions in a force field analysis?
    a. "What do you hope to accomplish in the meeting?"
    b. "What was bad about the meeting?"
    c. "What was good about the meeting?"
    d. "How can we improve meetings in the future?"

30. According to Title II of the Health Insurance and Portability and Accountability Act, disclosure of protected health information related to which of the following actions requires the patient's express written authorization?
    a. State in which the treatment occurred
    b. Health care operations
    c. Treatment
    d. Payment

31. Where does research suggest that the largest proportion of adverse events attributable to negligence occurs?
    a. Post-trauma unit
    b. Surgery unit
    c. Maternity ward
    d. Emergency room

32. Root cause analyses most often reveal that mistakes are the result of
    a. a series of small errors.
    b. a single miscalculation.
    c. a culture of incompetence.
    d. bad actors.

33. According to JCAHO, what is the primary cause of wrong-site surgery errors?
    a. Unusual patient characteristics
    b. The necessity of multiple surgeries
    c. Communication failure
    d. The presence of multiple surgeons

34. Why is it is easy to conduct a survey of medication-related errors?
    a. There are very few of these relative to other types of errors.
    b. Deaths caused by such errors are rarely discovered.
    c. Such errors have small but noticeable effects on health care costs.
    d. Prescription-drug use is common and well documented.

35. Which of the following pieces of information is available in the Health Care Integrity and Protection Data Bank but not the National Practitioner Data Bank?
    a. Medical malpractice payments
    b. Criminal convictions related to health care
    c. Loss of licensure
    d. Negative findings by a state certification authority

36. Which of the following is the source of the most medication errors?
    a. Orders that require lab results
    b. High-risk orders
    c. Automatic orders
    d. Verbal orders

37. A hospital manager notices that a significant proportion of medication errors in the facility involve the same two drugs. What is the most likely cause?
    a. The drugs are widely available.
    b. The drugs are made by the same company.
    c. The drugs come in similar packaging.
    d. The drugs are habit-forming.

38. Which of the following sentinel events is the most common?
    a. Criminal event
    b. Unintended retention of a foreign body
    c. Medication error
    d. Infection-related event

39. A hospital uses infusion pumps to deliver intravenous medications. However, these pumps occasionally malfunction, so a nurse is assigned to monitor their operation every so often. Is this a good strategy?
    a. No, because it depends on the vigilance of one employee.
    b. No, because it will distract the nurse from her other duties.
    c. Yes, because it makes one person directly responsible.
    d. Yes, because it gives the nurse a clear directive.

40. A doctor fails to administer an indicated test, and the patient's condition deteriorates to the point that he must be admitted to an inpatient facility. What is this an example of?
    a. Preventive error
    b. Treatment error
    c. Diagnostic error
    d. Communication error

41. Because the hospital is busy, an anesthesiologist is given less time than usual to examine the infusion device that will be delivering medication to a patient during surgery. The machine malfunctions, and the doctors on hand must work feverishly to save the patient's life. What is this an example of?
    a. Active error
    b. Equipment error
    c. System error
    d. Latent error

42. A hospital's medication system is vast, and various elements of it fall within the purview of several different departments. What is one important step toward reducing errors in this system?
    a. Make each department responsible for the system as a whole.
    b. Have each department use the same self-assessment tools.
    c. Give a single person responsibility for overseeing the entire system.
    d. Simplify it.

43. Which of the following conditions would NOT be classified as an emergency according to the Emergency Medical Treatment and Active Labor Act?
    a. Kidney failure
    b. Normal child labor
    c. Myocardial infarction
    d. Ruptured appendix

44. What does an adverse drug reaction do?
    a. Decreases the efficacy of therapy
    b. Increases the toxicity of other medication
    c. Both A and B
    d. Neither A nor B

45. What is the definitive proof of the success of a regulation program?
    a. Fewer complaints from customers
    b. A decreased need for inspections
    c. A boost in employee morale
    d. An increase in throughput

46. According to the Institute of Medicine, which of the following is NOT one of the domains of quality care?
    a. Government regulation
    b. Customization
    c. Safety
    d. Interventions consistent with the latest medical findings

47. The system limits of a process typically are based on the average and standard deviation of the
    a. yield and error rate.
    b. duration and validity.
    c. yield and duration.
    d. validity and yield.

48. In a typical hospital, approximately what percentage of errors is reported?
    a. Less than 5 percent
    b. Between 25 and 50 percent
    c. 75 percent
    d. Between 80 and 90 percent

49. What is the maximum penalty for Emergency Medical Treatment and Active Labor Act violations by a hospital with more than 100 beds?
   a. $50,000 per violation
   b. $100,000 per violation
   c. $500,000 per violation
   d. $1,000,000 per violation

50. In behavioral health, what is the most important sentinel event for root cause analysis?
   a. Discharge
   b. Death
   c. Recovery
   d. Medication error

Answers and Explanations

1. A: The four components of the SBAR situational briefing model are situation, background, assessment, and recommendation. This model for communication is used to organize the exchange of information during a crisis situation. The first step is to detail the situation. This is done by identifying oneself, one's position, and one's unit. Next, the health care employee should mention the patient's name and the room number to which the communication is referring. Finally, the employee should briefly describe the problem. The employee will then give background by identifying the relevant medical history, the treatment administered thus far, and the date of admission and admission diagnosis. The assessment component of situational briefing includes a description of any changes from previous assessments, as for instance with respect to pain, blood pressure rate, or mental status. Finally, the employee will offer a recommendation, as for instance that the patient needs to be seen by a physician or transferred to another unit.

2. C: The Patient Self-Determination Act does not give patients the right to select their medications. The Patient Self-Determination Act was established to give people more control over their health care, particularly at the end of life. The act gives people the right to refuse treatment, to assist in the decision-making process, and to make advance health directives (that is, directions for care should the person lose the ability to communicate or make decisions).

3. C: One advantage of a voluntary error reporting system over a mandatory reporting system is that voluntary systems elicit more reports from frontline practitioners. Research has consistently shown that doctors and nurses who work directly with patients are more likely to report errors when there is a voluntary system in place. Error reporting is a crucial area in quality improvement. An effective system is necessary for the acquisition of accurate data. At present, there is no standardized error-reporting system in health care, though there are several common models.

4. A: The process chain in a laboratory is particularly subject to variability. In most medical laboratories, there is a great degree of volatility in the number of samples. This can be devastating to efficiency, particularly as it can create delays or necessitate the hiring of extra employees. Many laboratories are adopting lean manufacturing strategies to reduce logjams and smooth out the variability of operations.

5. C: A root cause analysis of inpatient suicides would be most likely to discover problems with the physical environment. Staffing levels, staff orientation, and the availability of information also may contribute to suicide, but the physical environment is much more likely to be involved. Of course, most root cause analyses reveal that there are multiple factors involved in incidents of inpatient suicide.

6. B: Abuse is not one of the types of quality problems identified by the Institute of Medicine's National Roundtable on Health Care Quality. Misuse, overuse, and underuse are the three common problems; they also represent three sources of waste in health care. The National Roundtable on Health Care Quality was significant because it asserted that the provision of health care services can be assessed with scientific precision. This was a major step toward incorporating business and manufacturing productivity systems in health care.

7. C: In order for a patient to no longer be deserving of service under the Emergency Medical Treatment and Active Labor Act, he must be alert. The EMTALA requires hospitals to provide emergency care regardless of the ability to pay. Any hospital that accepts payment from the Department of Health and Human Services or the Centers for Medicare and Medicaid Services is required to abide by the EMTALA. The other answer choices are slightly incorrect. A patient does not need to provide the contact information of a caretaker if he is capable of caring for himself. Also, the hospital may not be required to continue serving patients who can eat and communicate by using special equipment.

8. C: Independent contractors are the group least likely to report errors. In part, this is because they have the least personal interest in the success of the health care facility. Also, an independent contractor is more likely to view his employment as tenuous and is therefore more nervous about admitting mistakes. A system that explicitly avoids punishing those who report will improve the incidence of error reporting among independent contractors.

9. A: Hospitals that implement computerized provider order entry (CPOE) almost always see a decline in medication errors. CPOE is a standard program for automating medical instructions. Implementation of a CPOE program diminishes errors related to faulty transcription or unclear handwriting. These programs also simplify inventory and decrease delays in order completion. Perhaps more importantly, in large facilities, the implementation of a CPOE program enables employees to give and receive orders without being in physical proximity to one another.

10. C: Whenever possible, medication orders should be by dose. This is the most important variable related to medication and the one that has the most relevance to the products actually used by the patient. Medication orders that are classified by weight, volume, or strength are often confusing to pharmacists. Moreover, several different unit systems (e.g., metric, SI) may be used, so there is a greater risk of error. To reduce the possibility of mistakes, health care facilities should standardize the protocol for medication orders.

11. C: When a hospital official notes that most errors are occurring at the "sharp end," he means that they occur during the interactions between caregivers and patients. The phrases *sharp end* and *blunt end* are used by quality management professionals to describe areas of practice. The sharp end is all of the operations that involve direct contact with the patient, client, or customer. The blunt end is all of the behind-the-scenes actions that take place outside of the awareness of the patient, client, or customer. Although patients are more likely to notice errors at the sharp end, there are significantly more errors committed at the blunt end.

12. D: Research suggests that people make fewer errors when they work in a team. There are a few reasons for this. For one thing, the desire to demonstrate competency in front of peers encourages people to attend more fully to their tasks. Also, the members of a group are able to correct one another. People do tend to make more errors when they work creatively, although these errors often lead to insight and innovation. Multitasking, however, increases the likelihood of error without providing any benefit. Research consistently shows that people who perform more than one task at the same time are less successful at each of the tasks.

13. D: State agencies may request information from the Health Care Integrity and Protection Data Bank. The other groups that may request information from this data bank are federal government agencies, health plans, health care practitioners, and researchers. However, researchers are only allowed to obtain statistical data from the data bank.

14. D: The cost of controls is not included in a calculation of risk priority number. A risk priority number, or RPN, is an objective picture of the importance of a particular danger to performance. It is calculated by rating on a scale from 1 to 10 the severity of each possible adverse effect (10 is the most severe), the likelihood of each of these effects (10 is the most certain to occur), and the effectiveness of possible controls (1 is the most effective), and then multiplying these three numbers.

15. D: A hemolytic transfusion reaction caused by blood group incompatibility would be defined as a *sentinel event* by the Joint Commission. In general, sentinel events are defined as any "unexpected occurrences involving death or serious physical or psychological injury, or the risk thereof." A hemolytic transfusion reaction caused by blood group incompatibility would be considered a sentinel event even if the patient does not die or suffer major permanent loss of function. Mistakes related to radiation therapy are considered sentinel events if therapy is delivered to the wrong region of the body or is at least 25 percent greater than the planned dose. Suicide is a sentinel event if it occurs in a continuous care setting or within three days of discharge. Neonatal jaundice is considered a sentinel event if it is severe (that is, if bilirubin is more than 30 mg/dl).

16. C: Before conducting a safety audit in an emergency department, an administrator first needs to obtain a written set of safety standards. This is necessary so that the administrator can compare his observations to the established protocol. The general purpose of a safety audit is to identify areas in which the department deviates from standard procedure. In order to perform an effective audit, the administrator needs to have a general familiarity with the rules that have been taught to his current employees.

17. C: In this scenario, the prescription should not count toward the pharmacy's yield. In lean service provision, only those processes that are completed without the necessity of reworking or repair are considered as a part of yield. The goal of lean service implementation is to improve yields by reducing errors and defects. Mistakes due to bad handwriting are common in health care, which has led many facilities to standardize notation and introduce labeling or bar coding systems. Such errors do not need to be reported to the FDA.

18. A: Federal agencies report information to the Health Care Integrity and Protection Data Bank. The other answer choices are groups that report information to the National Practitioner Data Bank. Health plans and state agencies are also required to report information to the Health Care Integrity and Protection Data Bank. The National Practitioner Data Bank also receives reports from professional societies with formal peer review, peer-review organizations, HMOs, group practices, managed care organizations, and state health care licensing and certification authorities.

19. B: In general, a failure modes and effects analysis (FMEA) should proceed two steps in each direction. A failure modes and effects analysis is a two-part process: identification of errors or defects (failure modes) and consideration of the consequences (effects analysis). After identifying the causes of error or defect, an FMEA might go on to identify the causes of

the causes. However, proceeding too far down this path can be fruitless. In the same way, evaluating the consequences of the consequences of failure can be productive, but to continue in this direction ultimately generates too much noise to be useful. In some cases, it will be productive to extend FMEA for more than two steps.

20. C: The Healthcare Quality Improvement Act provides confidentiality and legal immunity for health care peer-review processes to encourage participation by physicians. When the law was being drafted, the American Medical Association argued that, without these conditions, professionals would be reluctant to cooperate.

21. B: The first and most important step in a disclosure conversation is admitting error and apologizing. The wisdom of apologizing has long been a source of contention in health care circles. For many years, it was widely thought that an apology would leave the practitioner vulnerable to malpractice suits. However, recent legislation has established that apology does not equal an admission of negligence or malpractice. It is now considered prudent to mollify a potentially confrontational patient or client by issuing a sincere apology.

22. A: If an at-risk patient is left unattended and has an adverse response to medication, this is known as a *sentinel event*. A sentinel event is an adverse occurrence that is not in the normal progression of a patient's illness. The death of a patient from lung cancer would not be considered a sentinel event, for example. However, an adverse drug event is considered a sentinel event even if the patient is considered to be at risk. Whenever a sentinel event occurs, the health care facility should perform a root cause analysis.

23. D: The frequency of errors in a particular process would best be displayed in a histogram. Histograms are charts that display the frequencies of various events. It looks a bit like a bar chart, but the bars have varying widths depending on the magnitude of the frequency. A matrix diagram illustrates the relationships between multiple sets of data. A Pareto chart combines a bar graph with a line chart: The bar graph depicts frequencies in descending order, while the line graph illustrates the cumulative total. An affinity diagram illustrates the connections and similarities between items in a set of information.

24. C: A negative binomial distribution could be used to determine the number of blood transfusions that are likely to be performed before an error is made. Negative binomial distributions are effective for indicating how many successful events are likely to occur before a failure. This sort of statistical calculation is useful for monitoring trends in errors.

25. D: The scenario described in question 25 is an example of extra processing. Extra processing is anathema to the philosophy of lean. Whenever a lean manager spots a situation like the one described in question 25, he will immediately work to resolve it. In this case, the hospital would be wise to adopt a labeling system that is appropriate for all of its containers. Besides the obvious creation of more work, the extra processing described in this question may encourage medication errors.

26. B: An analysis of the root causes of an abnormally high number of restraint deaths is most likely to indicate problems with staff orientation and training. Equipment, staffing levels, and alarm systems can also be culpable in restraint deaths, but problems with orientation and training are much more likely. Restraint equipment has been designed to be very safe so long as it is used correctly. When used improperly, restraint equipment can be

deadly. It should be noted that most root cause analyses indicate problems in multiple areas.

27. D: The physical theft of data is responsible for the most privacy violations of the Health Insurance Portability and Accountability Act. Indeed, more than half of all privacy violations are related to the physical theft of data. The second-most common cause of privacy violations is disclosure without the authorization of the patient.

28. D: When it is impossible for medications to be standardized, it is important to differentiate them clearly. Many medications have similar packaging and labeling, and so, in order to reduce medication errors, they should be clearly distinguished. Hospitals and health care facilities often use color-coding or electronic tags to differentiate similar-looking medications.

29. A: "What do you hope to accomplish in the meeting?" is not one of the typical questions in a force field analysis. A force field analysis is a retrospective rather than a prospective look at meeting structure and organization. In other words, it is a tool used to review what has happened in the past rather than to plan for the future. Force field analysis is based on the idea that progress can be made by enumerating the forces that contribute to or hinder the achievement of goals. Facilitators often use this technique to streamline meetings.

30. A: According to Title II of the Health Insurance Portability and Accountability Act, disclosure of protected health information related to the state in which the treatment occurred requires the patient's express written authorization. The Health Insurance Portability and Accountability Act declares that certain categories of information must be treated with special care. Besides the information listed in the other answer choices, HIPAA designates as protected health information all names, geographic indicators smaller than a state, dates, phone numbers, e-mail addresses, Social Security numbers, driver's license numbers, IP addresses, biometric identifiers, photos, and other unique identifiers.

31. D: Research suggests that the largest proportion of adverse effects attributable to negligence occur in the emergency room. Of course, the volatile workload and elevated stress level of the emergency room is conducive to negligence. However, there are steps that can be taken to reduce these adverse events. Standardization and comprehensive training can diminish, though not eliminate, the incidence of adverse events related to negligence.

32. A: Root cause analyses most often reveal that mistakes are the result of a series of small errors. Moreover, mistakes and system failures are likely to be predicated on a series of small, often latent errors. This is one reason why it is impossible for frontline practitioners to eradicate errors through diligence and great effort. It is instead necessary for administrators and quality improvement managers to examine processes in their totality and eliminate sources of error.

33. C: According to JCAHO, the primary cause of wrong-site surgery errors is communication failure. Specifically, these errors are caused by incoherent or incomplete communication among practitioners. Communication factors can be caused by any number of external factors: noisy work environment, lack of a standardized notation system, or bad handwriting.

34. D: It is easy to conduct a survey of medication-related errors because prescription drug use is common and well documented. For this reason, there is vast literature on the subject. However, many other types of errors remain relatively unexplored. For instance, latent errors related to poor training or improper calibration of equipment are much less likely to be analyzed. Nevertheless, it is important to continue analyzing medication-related errors, both because they are quite common and because they are dangerous and costly. There is currently a movement to establish a standardized medication error-reporting system that will enable the compilation of statistics on a larger scale.

35. B: Criminal convictions related to health care are available in the Health Care Integrity and Protection Data Bank but not the National Practitioner Data Bank. The Health Care Integrity and Protection Data Bank and the National Practitioner Data Bank are the two main components of the federal health data bank. In addition to criminal convictions related to health care, the Health Care Integrity and Protection Data Bank also includes licensing and certification actions, exclusions from federal or state health care programs, and other adjudicated actions or decisions. In addition to the information described in the other answer choices, the National Practitioner Data Bank includes other adverse licensure actions, adverse clinical privileging actions; adverse professional society membership actions, negative actions by a peer-review organization, and negative actions by a private accreditation organization.

36. D: Verbal orders are the source of the most medication errors. Automatic orders, on the other hand, are responsible for the least medication errors. Verbal orders are more likely to be misunderstood or forgotten. Even though doctors have notoriously bad handwriting, written prescriptions are more likely to be filled correctly. It is best to automate prescriptions as much as possible and then to standardize the process for verbal orders. For instance, many facilities reduce errors by mandating that verbal prescriptions always be measured in metric units.

37. C: In the scenario described in question 37, the most likely cause is that the drugs come in similar packaging. Errors resulting from similar packaging are surprisingly common in health care facilities. Many facilities therefore take specific steps to label or otherwise differentiate such medications. Although it can be valuable to have standardized packaging for drugs, there must also be a clear and universal system for differentiation.

38. B: Of the given sentinel events, those related to the unintended retention of a foreign body are the most common. Other very common sentinel events are suicide, severe neonatal hyperbilirubinemia, post-op complications, and events in which the wrong patient or site is treated or in which the wrong procedure is used.

39. A: This is a bad strategy because it depends on the vigilance of one employee. Even the best employees will make mistakes, forget things, or lose their concentration. Important processes should never rely on a person to repeatedly remember to perform a task. Instead, there should be an automatic alert system that reminds multiple employees that a task needs to be performed.

40. C: When a doctor fails to administer an indicated test and the patient has an adverse result, the doctor has committed a diagnostic error. A diagnostic error has been committed whenever a condition is misidentified or an indicated test is not performed. Diagnostic errors can result in even more errors in the future. A preventive error is a mistaken

approach to avoiding a condition, while a treatment error is a mistake related to the resolution of a condition. Communication error may occur among service providers or among service providers and patients.

41. D: The scenario described in question 41 is an example of latent error. A latent error is one made during setup or programming, which creates negative consequences in the future. These sorts of errors are very difficult to identify because they take place far removed from the adverse events. In question 41, latent error is present both in the malfunction of the machine and the paucity of time allotted to the anesthesiologist. Many times, it takes a combination of latent errors to create an adverse event. Hospital managers are responsible for taking a detached and broad view of operations to identify and eliminate the sources of latent error.

42. C: One important step toward reducing errors in a system that spans several departments is giving a single person responsibility for overseeing the entire system. Often, the sources of error can be spotted only when a single person examines the system as a whole. It may be impossible for one person to examine the system in every area in detail, but a general supervisor may be able to spot areas in which departments are performing the same functions differently. This sort of inconsistency can lead to errors that may be impossible for department heads, with their limited view, to see.

43. B: Normal child labor would not be classified as an emergency according to the Emergency Medical Treatment and Active Labor Act. If the health of the mother or of the unborn child is endangered, then child labor may be classified as an emergency. In such a case, the emergency is considered to continue until the child is delivered. All of the other answer choices are conditions that would be considered emergencies under the EMTALA. In general, a condition is defined as an emergency when it appears with symptoms that are severe enough to place the health of the patient in jeopardy or when it impairs bodily organs or functions.

44. C: An adverse drug reaction decreases the efficacy of therapy and increases the toxicity of other medication. It should be stressed that an adverse drug reaction occurs in response to a normal dose of medication. Overdoses are defined differently. Health care facilities need to have a standard process for evaluating and cataloging adverse drug reactions, so they can develop policies to reduce them.

45. B: The definitive proof of the success of a regulation program is a decreased need for inspections. Ultimately, the presence of a comprehensive and effective regulatory system means that rules are followed without enforcement being required as often. The other answer choices represent frequent positive consequences of effective regulation but are not necessarily indicative of regulatory success. The initial costs of implementing a regulatory program can be high, but in the long run, such measures are cost-effective.

46. A: According to the Institute of Medicine, the three domains of quality care are customization, safety, and interventions consistent with the latest medical findings. These domains provide the basic structure for the IOM's recommendations about quality care, originally presented in the groundbreaking book *To Err Is Human*. Government regulation is an essential part of quality care, but it is not a domain in itself. Instead, the IOM recommends that health care facilities work with government agencies to develop fair but efficient regulatory policies that protect practitioners and patients alike.

47. C: The system limits of a process typically are based on the average and standard deviation of the yield and duration. That is, the system can only be expected to perform within the measured ranges of quantity produced and time of operation. The intention of Six Sigma is to improve the yield and duration and thereby the system limits.

48. A: In a typical hospital, less than 5 percent of errors are reported. Many hospital managers are surprised by this statistic because the number of reported errors can seem large. However, health care facilities often have unclear or relaxed reporting policies. Part-time employees and independent contractors are much less likely to report errors. Unfortunately, the failure to report errors has negative consequences far beyond the point at which the specific error occurs. The best health care facilities establish mandatory error-reporting programs, with an emphasis on being nonjudgmental and accepting of inevitable human error.

49. A: The maximum penalty for Emergency Medical Treatment and Active Labor Act violations by a hospital with more than 100 beds is $50,000 per violation. Hospitals that have fewer than 100 beds are subject to maximum fines of only $25,000. Individual physicians are subject to fines of $50,000 per violation.

50. B: In behavioral health, the most important sentinel event for root cause analysis is death. A sentinel event is any adverse occurrence that is outside the range of the normal progression of the diagnosed illness. In other words, death can only be a sentinel event when it occurs in patients who are not expected to die. In cases where death is not considered likely, it is usually the most important sentinel event because it is the one that most urgently requires investigation and prevention. The term *sentinel event* was popularized by the Joint Commission on Accreditation of Healthcare Organizations.

Secret Key #1 - Time is Your Greatest Enemy

Pace Yourself

Wear a watch. At the beginning of the test, check the time (or start a chronometer on your watch to count the minutes), and check the time after every few questions to make sure you are "on schedule."

If you are forced to speed up, do it efficiently. Usually one or more answer choices can be eliminated without too much difficulty. Above all, don't panic. Don't speed up and just begin guessing at random choices. By pacing yourself, and continually monitoring your progress against your watch, you will always know exactly how far ahead or behind you are with your available time. If you find that you are one minute behind on the test, don't skip one question without spending any time on it, just to catch back up. Take 15 fewer seconds on the next four questions, and after four questions you'll have caught back up. Once you catch back up, you can continue working each problem at your normal pace.

Furthermore, don't dwell on the problems that you were rushed on. If a problem was taking up too much time and you made a hurried guess, it must be difficult. The difficult questions are the ones you are most likely to miss anyway, so it isn't a big loss. It is better to end with more time than you need than to run out of time.

Lastly, sometimes it is beneficial to slow down if you are constantly getting ahead of time. You are always more likely to catch a careless mistake by working more slowly than quickly, and among very high-scoring test takers (those who are likely to have lots of time left over), careless errors affect the score more than mastery of material.

Secret Key #2 - Guessing is not Guesswork

You probably know that guessing is a good idea. Unlike other standardized tests, there is no penalty for getting a wrong answer. Even if you have no idea about a question, you still have a 20-25% chance of getting it right.

Most test takers do not understand the impact that proper guessing can have on their score. Unless you score extremely high, guessing will significantly contribute to your final score.

Monkeys Take the Test

What most test takers don't realize is that to insure that 20-25% chance, you have to guess randomly. If you put 20 monkeys in a room to take this test, assuming they answered once per question and behaved themselves, on average they would get 20-25% of the questions correct. Put 20 test takers in the room, and the average will be much lower among guessed questions. Why?

1. The test writers intentionally write deceptive answer choices that "look" right. A test taker has no idea about a question, so he picks the "best looking" answer, which is often wrong. The monkey has no idea what looks good and what doesn't, so it will consistently be right about 20-25% of the time.
2. Test takers will eliminate answer choices from the guessing pool based on a hunch or intuition. Simple but correct answers often get excluded, leaving a 0% chance of being correct. The monkey has no clue, and often gets lucky with the best choice.

This is why the process of elimination endorsed by most test courses is flawed and detrimental to your performance. Test takers don't guess; they make an ignorant stab in the dark that is usually worse than random.

$5 Challenge

Let me introduce one of the most valuable ideas of this course—the $5 challenge:

You only mark your "best guess" if you are willing to bet $5 on it.
You only eliminate choices from guessing if you are willing to bet $5 on it.

Why $5? Five dollars is an amount of money that is small yet not insignificant, and can really add up fast (20 questions could cost you $100). Likewise, each answer choice on one question of the test will have a small impact on your overall score, but it can really add up to a lot of points in the end.

The process of elimination IS valuable. The following shows your chance of guessing it right:

If you eliminate wrong answer choices until only this many remain:	Chance of getting it correct:
1	100%
2	50%
3	33%

However, if you accidentally eliminate the right answer or go on a hunch for an incorrect answer, your chances drop dramatically—to 0%. By guessing among all the answer choices, you are GUARANTEED to have a shot at the right answer.

That's why the $5 test is so valuable. If you give up the advantage and safety of a pure guess, it had better be worth the risk.

What we still haven't covered is how to be sure that whatever guess you make is truly random. Here's the easiest way:

Always pick the first answer choice among those remaining.

Such a technique means that you have decided, **before you see a single test question**, exactly how you are going to guess, and since the order of choices tells you nothing about which one is correct, this guessing technique is perfectly random.

This section is not meant to scare you away from making educated guesses or eliminating choices; you just need to define when a choice is worth eliminating. The $5 test, along with a pre-defined random guessing strategy, is the best way to make sure you reap all of the benefits of guessing.

Secret Key #3 - Practice Smarter, Not Harder

Many test takers delay the test preparation process because they dread the awful amounts of practice time they think necessary to succeed on the test. We have refined an effective method that will take you only a fraction of the time.

There are a number of "obstacles" in the path to success. Among these are answering questions, finishing in time, and mastering test-taking strategies. All must be executed on the day of the test at peak performance, or your score will suffer. The test is a mental marathon that has a large impact on your future.

Just like a marathon runner, it is important to work your way up to the full challenge. So first you just worry about questions, and then time, and finally strategy:

Success Strategy

1. Find a good source for practice tests.
2. If you are willing to make a larger time investment, consider using more than one study guide. Often the different approaches of multiple authors will help you "get" difficult concepts.
3. Take a practice test with no time constraints, with all study helps, "open book." Take your time with questions and focus on applying strategies.
4. Take a practice test with time constraints, with all guides, "open book."
5. Take a final practice test without open material and with time limits.

If you have time to take more practice tests, just repeat step 5. By gradually exposing yourself to the full rigors of the test environment, you will condition your mind to the stress of test day and maximize your success.

Secret Key #4 - Prepare, Don't Procrastinate

Let me state an obvious fact: if you take the test three times, you will probably get three different scores. This is due to the way you feel on test day, the level of preparedness you have, and the version of the test you see. Despite the test writers' claims to the contrary, some versions of the test WILL be easier for you than others.

Since your future depends so much on your score, you should maximize your chances of success. In order to maximize the likelihood of success, you've got to prepare in advance. This means taking practice tests and spending time learning the information and test taking strategies you will need to succeed.

Never go take the actual test as a "practice" test, expecting that you can just take it again if you need to. Take all the practice tests you can on your own, but when you go to take the official test, be prepared, be focused, and do your best the first time!

Secret Key #5 - Test Yourself

Everyone knows that time is money. There is no need to spend too much of your time or too little of your time preparing for the test. You should only spend as much of your precious time preparing as is necessary for you to get the score you need.

Once you have taken a practice test under real conditions of time constraints, then you will know if you are ready for the test or not.

If you have scored extremely high the first time that you take the practice test, then there is not much point in spending countless hours studying. You are already there.

Benchmark your abilities by retaking practice tests and seeing how much you have improved. Once you consistently score high enough to guarantee success, then you are ready.

If you have scored well below where you need, then knuckle down and begin studying in earnest. Check your improvement regularly through the use of practice tests under real conditions. Above all, don't worry, panic, or give up. The key is perseverance!

Then, when you go to take the test, remain confident and remember how well you did on the practice tests. If you can score high enough on a practice test, then you can do the same on the real thing.

General Strategies

The most important thing you can do is to ignore your fears and jump into the test immediately. Do not be overwhelmed by any strange-sounding terms. You have to jump into the test like jumping into a pool—all at once is the easiest way.

Make Predictions

As you read and understand the question, try to guess what the answer will be. Remember that several of the answer choices are wrong, and once you begin reading them, your mind will immediately become cluttered with answer choices designed to throw you off. Your mind is typically the most focused immediately after you have read the question and digested its contents. If you can, try to predict what the correct answer will be. You may be surprised at what you can predict.

Quickly scan the choices and see if your prediction is in the listed answer choices. If it is, then you can be quite confident that you have the right answer. It still won't hurt to check the other answer choices, but most of the time, you've got it!

Answer the Question

It may seem obvious to only pick answer choices that answer the question, but the test writers can create some excellent answer choices that are wrong. Don't pick an answer just because it sounds right, or you believe it to be true. It MUST answer the question. Once you've made your selection, always go back and check it against the question and make sure that you didn't misread the question and that the answer choice does answer the question posed.

Benchmark

After you read the first answer choice, decide if you think it sounds correct or not. If it doesn't, move on to the next answer choice. If it does, mentally mark that answer choice. This doesn't mean that you've definitely selected it as your answer choice, it just means that it's the best you've seen thus far. Go ahead and read the next choice. If the next choice is worse than the one you've already selected, keep going to the next answer choice. If the next choice is better than the choice you've already selected, mentally mark the new answer choice as your best guess.

The first answer choice that you select becomes your standard. Every other answer choice must be benchmarked against that standard. That choice is correct until proven otherwise by another answer choice beating it out. Once you've decided that no other answer choice seems as good, do one final check to ensure that your answer choice answers the question posed.

Valid Information

Don't discount any of the information provided in the question. Every piece of information may be necessary to determine the correct answer. None of the information in the question is there to throw you off (while the answer choices will certainly have information to throw you off). If two seemingly unrelated topics are discussed, don't ignore either. You can be confident there is a relationship, or it wouldn't be included in the question, and you are probably going to have to determine what is that relationship to find the answer.

Avoid "Fact Traps"

Don't get distracted by a choice that is factually true. Your search is for the answer that answers the question. Stay focused and don't fall for an answer that is true but irrelevant. Always go back to the question and make sure you're choosing an answer that actually answers the question and is not just a true statement. An answer can be factually correct, but it MUST answer the question asked. Additionally, two answers can both be seemingly correct, so be sure to read all of the answer choices, and make sure that you get the one that BEST answers the question.

Milk the Question

Some of the questions may throw you completely off. They might deal with a subject you have not been exposed to, or one that you haven't reviewed in years. While your lack of knowledge about the subject will be a hindrance, the question itself can give you many clues that will help you find the correct answer. Read the question carefully and look for clues. Watch particularly for adjectives and nouns describing difficult terms or words that you don't recognize. Regardless of whether you completely understand a word or not, replacing it with a synonym, either provided or one you more familiar with, may help you to understand what the questions are asking. Rather than wracking your mind about specific detailed information concerning a difficult term or word, try to use mental substitutes that are easier to understand.

The Trap of Familiarity

Don't just choose a word because you recognize it. On difficult questions, you may not recognize a number of words in the answer choices. The test writers don't put "make-believe" words on the test, so don't think that just because you only recognize all the words in one answer choice that that answer choice must be correct. If you only recognize words in one answer choice, then focus on that one. Is it correct? Try your best to determine if it is correct. If it is, that's great. If not, eliminate it. Each word and answer choice you eliminate increases your chances of getting the question correct, even if you then have to guess among the unfamiliar choices.

Eliminate Answers

Eliminate choices as soon as you realize they are wrong. But be careful! Make sure you consider all of the possible answer choices. Just because one appears right, doesn't mean that the next one won't be even better! The test writers will usually put more than one good answer choice for every question, so read all of them. Don't worry if you are stuck between two that seem right. By getting down to just two remaining possible choices, your odds are now 50/50. Rather than wasting too much time, play the odds. You are guessing, but guessing wisely because you've been able to knock out some of the answer choices that you know are wrong. If you are eliminating choices and realize that the last answer choice you are left with is also obviously wrong, don't panic. Start over and consider each choice again. There may easily be something that you missed the first time and will realize on the second pass.

Tough Questions

If you are stumped on a problem or it appears too hard or too difficult, don't waste time. Move on! Remember though, if you can quickly check for obviously incorrect answer choices, your chances of guessing correctly are greatly improved. Before you completely give up, at least try to knock out a couple of possible answers. Eliminate what you can and then guess at the remaining answer choices before moving on.

Brainstorm

If you get stuck on a difficult question, spend a few seconds quickly brainstorming. Run through the complete list of possible answer choices. Look at each choice and ask yourself, "Could this answer the question satisfactorily?" Go through each answer choice and consider it independently of the others. By systematically going through all possibilities, you may find something that you would otherwise overlook. Remember though that when you get stuck, it's important to try to keep moving.

Read Carefully

Understand the problem. Read the question and answer choices carefully. Don't miss the question because you misread the terms. You have plenty of time to read each question thoroughly and make sure you understand what is being asked. Yet a happy medium must be attained, so don't waste too much time. You must read carefully, but efficiently.

Face Value

When in doubt, use common sense. Always accept the situation in the problem at face value. Don't read too much into it. These problems will not require you to make huge leaps of logic. The test writers aren't trying to throw you off with a cheap trick. If you have to go beyond creativity and make a leap of logic in order to have an answer choice answer the question, then you should look at the other answer choices. Don't overcomplicate the problem by creating theoretical relationships or explanations that will warp time or space. These are normal problems rooted in reality. It's just that the applicable relationship or explanation may not be readily apparent and you have to figure things out. Use your common sense to interpret anything that isn't clear.

Prefixes

If you're having trouble with a word in the question or answer choices, try dissecting it. Take advantage of every clue that the word might include. Prefixes and suffixes can be a huge help. Usually they allow you to determine a basic meaning. Pre- means before, post- means after, pro - is positive, de- is negative. From these prefixes and suffixes, you can get an idea of the general meaning of the word and try to put it into context. Beware though of any traps. Just because con- is the opposite of pro-, doesn't necessarily mean congress is the opposite of progress!

Hedge Phrases

Watch out for critical hedge phrases, led off with words such as "likely," "may," "can," "sometimes," "often," "almost," "mostly," "usually," "generally," "rarely," and "sometimes." Question writers insert these hedge phrases to cover every possibility. Often an answer choice will be wrong simply because it leaves no room for exception. Unless the situation calls for them, avoid answer choices that have definitive words like "exactly," and "always."

Switchback Words

Stay alert for "switchbacks." These are the words and phrases frequently used to alert you to shifts in thought. The most common switchback word is "but." Others include "although," "however," "nevertheless," "on the other hand," "even though," "while," "in spite of," "despite," and "regardless of."

New Information

Correct answer choices will rarely have completely new information included. Answer choices typically are straightforward reflections of the material asked about and will directly relate to the question. If a new piece of information is included in an answer choice that doesn't even seem to relate to the topic being asked about, then that answer choice is likely incorrect. All of the information needed to answer the question is usually provided for you in the question. You should not have to make guesses that are unsupported or choose answer choices that require unknown information that cannot be reasoned from what is given.

Time Management

On technical questions, don't get lost on the technical terms. Don't spend too much time on any one question. If you don't know what a term means, then odds are you aren't going to get much further since you don't have a dictionary. You should be able to immediately recognize whether or not you know a term. If you don't, work with the other clues that you have—the other answer choices and terms provided—but don't waste too much time trying to figure out a difficult term that you don't know.

Contextual Clues

Look for contextual clues. An answer can be right but not the correct answer. The contextual clues will help you find the answer that is most right and is correct. Understand the context in which a phrase or statement is made. This will help you make important distinctions.

Don't Panic

Panicking will not answer any questions for you; therefore, it isn't helpful. When you first see the question, if your mind goes blank, take a deep breath. Force yourself to mechanically go through the steps of solving the problem using the strategies you've learned.

Pace Yourself

Don't get clock fever. It's easy to be overwhelmed when you're looking at a page full of questions, your mind is full of random thoughts and feeling confused, and the clock is ticking down faster than you would like. Calm down and maintain the pace that you have set for yourself. As long as you are on track by monitoring your pace, you are guaranteed to have enough time for yourself. When you get to the last few minutes of the test, it may seem like you won't have enough time left, but if you only have as many questions as you should have left at that point, then you're right on track!

Answer Selection

The best way to pick an answer choice is to eliminate all of those that are wrong, until only one is left and confirm that is the correct answer. Sometimes though, an answer choice may immediately look right. Be careful! Take a second to make sure that the other choices are not equally obvious. Don't make a hasty mistake. There are only two times that you should stop before checking other answers. First is when you are positive that the answer choice you have selected is correct. Second is when time is almost out and you have to make a quick guess!

Check Your Work

Since you will probably not know every term listed and the answer to every question, it is important that you get credit for the ones that you do know. Don't miss any questions through careless mistakes. If at all possible, try to take a second to look back over your answer selection and make sure you've selected the correct answer choice and haven't made a costly careless mistake (such as marking an answer choice that you didn't mean to mark). The time it takes for this quick double check should more than pay for itself in caught mistakes.

Beware of Directly Quoted Answers

Sometimes an answer choice will repeat word for word a portion of the question or reference section. However, beware of such exact duplication. It may be a trap! More than likely, the correct choice will paraphrase or summarize a point, rather than being exactly the same wording.

Slang

Scientific sounding answers are better than slang ones. An answer choice that begins "To compare the outcomes..." is much more likely to be correct than one that begins "Because some people insisted..."

Extreme Statements

Avoid wild answers that throw out highly controversial ideas that are proclaimed as established fact. An answer choice that states the "process should used in certain situations, if..." is much more likely to be correct than one that states the "process should be discontinued completely." The first is a calm rational statement and doesn't even make a definitive, uncompromising stance, using a hedge word "if" to provide wiggle room, whereas the second choice is a radical idea and far more extreme.

Answer Choice Families

When you have two or more answer choices that are direct opposites or parallels, one of them is usually the correct answer. For instance, if one answer choice states "x increases" and another answer choice states "x decreases" or "y increases," then those two or three answer choices are very similar in construction and fall into the same family of answer choices. A family of answer choices consists of two or three answer choices, very similar in construction, but often with directly opposite meanings. Usually the correct answer choice will be in that family of answer choices. The "odd man out" or answer choice that doesn't seem to fit the parallel construction of the other answer choices is more likely to be incorrect.

Special Report: How to Overcome Test Anxiety

The very nature of tests caters to some level of anxiety, nervousness, or tension, just as we feel for any important event that occurs in our lives. A little bit of anxiety or nervousness can be a good thing. It helps us with motivation, and makes achievement just that much sweeter. However, too much anxiety can be a problem, especially if it hinders our ability to function and perform.

"Test anxiety," is the term that refers to the emotional reactions that some test-takers experience when faced with a test or exam. Having a fear of testing and exams is based upon a rational fear, since the test-taker's performance can shape the course of an academic career. Nevertheless, experiencing excessive fear of examinations will only interfere with the test-taker's ability to perform and chance to be successful.

There are a large variety of causes that can contribute to the development and sensation of test anxiety. These include, but are not limited to, lack of preparation and worrying about issues surrounding the test.

Lack of Preparation

Lack of preparation can be identified by the following behaviors or situations:

Not scheduling enough time to study, and therefore cramming the night before the test or exam
Managing time poorly, to create the sensation that there is not enough time to do everything
Failing to organize the text information in advance, so that the study material consists of the entire text and not simply the pertinent information
Poor overall studying habits

Worrying, on the other hand, can be related to both the test taker, or many other factors around him/her that will be affected by the results of the test. These include worrying about:

Previous performances on similar exams, or exams in general
How friends and other students are achieving
The negative consequences that will result from a poor grade or failure

There are three primary elements to test anxiety. Physical components, which involve the same typical bodily reactions as those to acute anxiety (to be discussed below). Emotional factors have to do with fear or panic. Mental or cognitive issues concerning attention spans and memory abilities.

Physical Signals

There are many different symptoms of test anxiety, and these are not limited to mental and emotional strain. Frequently there are a range of physical signals that will let a test taker know that he/she is suffering from test anxiety. These bodily changes can include the following:

Perspiring
Sweaty palms
Wet, trembling hands
Nausea
Dry mouth
A knot in the stomach
Headache
Faintness
Muscle tension
Aching shoulders, back and neck
Rapid heart beat
Feeling too hot/cold

To recognize the sensation of test anxiety, a test-taker should monitor him/herself for the following sensations:

The physical distress symptoms as listed above
Emotional sensitivity, expressing emotional feelings such as the need to cry or laugh too much, or a sensation of anger or helplessness
A decreased ability to think, causing the test-taker to blank out or have racing thoughts that are hard to organize or control.

Though most students will feel some level of anxiety when faced with a test or exam, the majority can cope with that anxiety and maintain it at a manageable level. However, those who cannot are faced with a very real and very serious condition, which can and should be controlled for the immeasurable benefit of this sufferer.

Naturally, these sensations lead to negative results for the testing experience. The most common effects of test anxiety have to do with nervousness and mental blocking.

Nervousness

Nervousness can appear in several different levels:

The test-taker's difficulty, or even inability to read and understand the questions on the test
The difficulty or inability to organize thoughts to a coherent form
The difficulty or inability to recall key words and concepts relating to the testing questions (especially essays)
The receipt of poor grades on a test, though the test material was well known by the test taker

Conversely, a person may also experience mental blocking, which involves:

Blanking out on test questions
Only remembering the correct answers to the questions when the test has already finished.

Fortunately for test anxiety sufferers, beating these feelings, to a large degree, has to do with proper preparation. When a test taker has a feeling of preparedness, then anxiety will be dramatically lessened.

The first step to resolving anxiety issues is to distinguish which of the two types of anxiety are being suffered. If the anxiety is a direct result of a lack of preparation, this should be considered a normal reaction, and the anxiety level (as opposed to the test results) shouldn't be anything to worry about. However, if, when adequately prepared, the test-taker still panics, blanks out, or seems to overreact, this is not a fully rational reaction. While this can be considered normal too, there are many ways to combat and overcome these effects.

Remember that anxiety cannot be entirely eliminated, however, there are ways to minimize it, to make the anxiety easier to manage. Preparation is one of the best ways to minimize test anxiety. Therefore the following techniques are wise in order to best fight off any anxiety that may want to build.

To begin with, try to avoid cramming before a test, whenever it is possible. By trying to memorize an entire term's worth of information in one day, you'll be shocking your system, and not giving yourself a very good chance to absorb the information. This is an easy path to anxiety, so for those who suffer from test anxiety, cramming should not even be considered an option.

Instead of cramming, work throughout the semester to combine all of the material which is presented throughout the semester, and work on it gradually as the course goes by, making sure to master the main concepts first, leaving minor details for a week or so before the test.

To study for the upcoming exam, be sure to pose questions that may be on the examination, to gauge the ability to answer them by integrating the ideas from your texts, notes and lectures, as well as any supplementary readings.

If it is truly impossible to cover all of the information that was covered in that particular term, concentrate on the most important portions, that can be covered very well. Learn these concepts as best as possible, so that when the test comes, a goal can be made to use these concepts as presentations of your knowledge.

In addition to study habits, changes in attitude are critical to beating a struggle with test anxiety. In fact, an improvement of the perspective over the entire test-taking experience can actually help a test taker to enjoy studying and therefore improve the overall experience. Be certain not to overemphasize the significance of the grade - know that the result of the test is neither a reflection of self worth, nor is it a measure of intelligence; one grade will not predict a person's future success.

To improve an overall testing outlook, the following steps should be tried:

Keeping in mind that the most reasonable expectation for taking a test is to expect to try to demonstrate as much of what you know as you possibly can.
Reminding ourselves that a test is only one test; this is not the only one, and there will be others.
The thought of thinking of oneself in an irrational, all-or-nothing term should be avoided at all costs.
A reward should be designated for after the test, so there's something to look forward to. Whether it be going to a movie, going out to eat, or simply visiting friends, schedule it in advance, and do it no matter what result is expected on the exam.

Test-takers should also keep in mind that the basics are some of the most important things, even beyond anti-anxiety techniques and studying. Never neglect the basic social, emotional and biological needs, in order to try to absorb information. In order to best achieve, these three factors must be held as just as important as the studying itself.

Study Steps

Remember the following important steps for studying:

Maintain healthy nutrition and exercise habits. Continue both your recreational activities and social pass times. These both contribute to your physical and emotional well being.
Be certain to get a good amount of sleep, especially the night before the test, because when you're overtired you are not able to perform to the best of your best ability.
Keep the studying pace to a moderate level by taking breaks when they are needed, and varying the work whenever possible, to keep the mind fresh instead of getting bored.
When enough studying has been done that all the material that can be learned has been learned, and the test taker is prepared for the test, stop studying and do something relaxing such as listening to music, watching a movie, or taking a warm bubble bath.

There are also many other techniques to minimize the uneasiness or apprehension that is experienced along with test anxiety before, during, or even after the examination. In fact, there are a great deal of things that can be done to stop anxiety from interfering with lifestyle and performance. Again, remember that anxiety will not be eliminated entirely, and it shouldn't be. Otherwise that "up" feeling for exams would not exist, and most of us depend on that sensation to perform better than usual. However, this anxiety has to be at a level that is manageable.

Of course, as we have just discussed, being prepared for the exam is half the battle right away. Attending all classes, finding out what knowledge will be expected on the exam, and knowing the exam schedules are easy steps to lowering anxiety. Keeping up with work will remove the need to cram, and efficient study habits will eliminate wasted time. Studying should be done in an ideal location for concentration, so that it is simple to become interested in the material and give it complete attention. A method such as SQ3R (Survey, Question, Read, Recite, Review) is a wonderful key to follow to make sure that the study habits are as effective as possible, especially in the case of learning from a textbook. Flashcards are great techniques for memorization. Learning to take good notes will mean that notes will be full of useful information, so that less sifting will need to be done to seek out what is pertinent for studying. Reviewing notes after class and then again on occasion will keep the information fresh in the mind. From notes that have been taken summary sheets and outlines can be made for simpler reviewing.

A study group can also be a very motivational and helpful place to study, as there will be a sharing of ideas, all of the minds can work together, to make sure that everyone understands, and the studying will be made more interesting because it will be a social occasion.

Basically, though, as long as the test-taker remains organized and self confident, with efficient study habits, less time will need to be spent studying, and higher grades will be achieved.

To become self confident, there are many useful steps. The first of these is "self talk." It has been shown through extensive research, that self-talk for students who suffer from test anxiety, should be well monitored, in order to make sure that it contributes to self confidence as opposed to sinking the student. Frequently the self talk of test-anxious students is negative or self-defeating, thinking that everyone else is smarter and faster, that they always mess up, and that if they don't do well, they'll fail the entire course. It is important to decreasing anxiety that awareness is made of self talk. Try writing any negative self thoughts and then disputing them with a positive statement instead. Begin self-encouragement as though it was a friend speaking. Repeat positive statements to help reprogram the mind to believing in successes instead of failures.

Helpful Techniques

Other extremely helpful techniques include:

Self-visualization of doing well and reaching goals
While aiming for an "A" level of understanding, don't try to "overprotect" by setting your expectations lower. This will only convince the mind to stop studying in order to meet the lower expectations.
Don't make comparisons with the results or habits of other students. These are individual factors, and different things work for different people, causing different results.
Strive to become an expert in learning what works well, and what can be done in order to improve. Consider collecting this data in a journal.
Create rewards for after studying instead of doing things before studying that will only turn into avoidance behaviors.
Make a practice of relaxing - by using methods such as progressive relaxation, self-hypnosis, guided imagery, etc - in order to make relaxation an automatic sensation.
Work on creating a state of relaxed concentration so that concentrating will take on the focus of the mind, so that none will be wasted on worrying.
Take good care of the physical self by eating well and getting enough sleep.
Plan in time for exercise and stick to this plan.

Beyond these techniques, there are other methods to be used before, during and after the test that will help the test-taker perform well in addition to overcoming anxiety.

Before the exam comes the academic preparation. This involves establishing a study schedule and beginning at least one week before the actual date of the test. By doing this, the anxiety of not having enough time to study for the test will be automatically eliminated. Moreover, this will make the studying a much more effective experience, ensuring that the learning will be an easier process. This relieves much undue pressure on the test-taker.

Summary sheets, note cards, and flash cards with the main concepts and examples of these main concepts should be prepared in advance of the actual studying time. A topic should never be eliminated from this process. By omitting a topic because it isn't expected to be on the test is only setting up the test-taker for anxiety should it actually appear on the exam. Utilize the course syllabus for laying out the topics that should be studied. Carefully go over the notes that were made in class, paying special attention to any of the issues that the professor took special care to emphasize while lecturing in class. In the textbooks, use the chapter review, or if possible, the chapter tests, to begin your review.

It may even be possible to ask the instructor what information will be covered on the exam, or what the format of the exam will be (for example, multiple choice, essay, free form, true-false). Additionally, see if it is possible to find out how many questions will be on the test. If a review sheet or sample test has been offered by the professor, make good use of it, above anything else, for the preparation for the test. Another great resource for getting to know the examination is reviewing tests from previous semesters. Use these tests to review, and aim to achieve a 100% score on each of the possible topics. With a few exceptions, the goal that you set for yourself is the highest one that you will reach.

Take all of the questions that were assigned as homework, and rework them to any other possible course material. The more problems reworked, the more skill and confidence will form as a result. When forming the solution to a problem, write out each of the steps. Don't simply do head work. By doing as many steps on paper as possible, much clarification and therefore confidence will be formed. Do this with as many homework problems as possible, before checking the answers. By checking the answer after each problem, a reinforcement will exist, that will not be on the exam. Study situations should be as exam-like as possible, to prime the test-taker's system for the experience. By waiting to check the answers at the end, a psychological advantage will be formed, to decrease the stress factor.

Another fantastic reason for not cramming is the avoidance of confusion in concepts, especially when it comes to mathematics. 8-10 hours of study will become one hundred percent more effective if it is spread out over a week or at least several days, instead of doing it all in one sitting. Recognize that the human brain requires time in order to assimilate new material, so frequent breaks and a span of study time over several days will be much more beneficial.

Additionally, don't study right up until the point of the exam. Studying should stop a minimum of one hour before the exam begins. This allows the brain to rest and put things in their proper order. This will also provide the time to become as relaxed as possible when going into the examination room. The test-taker will also have time to eat well and eat sensibly. Know that the brain needs food as much as the rest of the body. With enough food and enough sleep, as well as a relaxed attitude, the body and the mind are primed for success.

Avoid any anxious classmates who are talking about the exam. These students only spread anxiety, and are not worth sharing the anxious sentimentalities.

Before the test also involves creating a positive attitude, so mental preparation should also be a point of concentration. There are many keys to creating a positive attitude. Should fears become rushing in, make a visualization of taking the exam, doing well, and seeing an A written on the paper. Write out a list of affirmations that will bring a feeling of confidence, such as "I am doing well in my English class," "I studied well and know my material," "I enjoy this class." Even if the affirmations aren't believed at first, it sends a positive message to the subconscious which will result in an alteration of the overall belief system, which is the system that creates reality.

If a sensation of panic begins, work with the fear and imagine the very worst! Work through the entire scenario of not passing the test, failing the entire course, and dropping out of school, followed by not getting a job, and pushing a shopping cart through the dark alley where you'll live. This will place things into perspective! Then, practice deep breathing and create a visualization of the opposite situation - achieving an "A" on the exam, passing the entire course, receiving the degree at a graduation ceremony.

On the day of the test, there are many things to be done to ensure the best results, as well as the most calm outlook. The following stages are suggested in order to maximize test-taking potential:

Begin the examination day with a moderate breakfast, and avoid any coffee or beverages with caffeine if the test taker is prone to jitters. Even people who are used to managing caffeine can feel jittery or light-headed when it is taken on a test day.
Attempt to do something that is relaxing before the examination begins. As last minute cramming clouds the mastering of overall concepts, it is better to use this time to create a calming outlook.
Be certain to arrive at the test location well in advance, in order to provide time to select a location that is away from doors, windows and other distractions, as well as giving enough time to relax before the test begins.
Keep away from anxiety generating classmates who will upset the sensation of stability and relaxation that is being attempted before the exam.
Should the waiting period before the exam begins cause anxiety, create a self-distraction by reading a light magazine or something else that is relaxing and simple.

During the exam itself, read the entire exam from beginning to end, and find out how much time should be allotted to each individual problem. Once writing the exam, should more time be taken for a problem, it should be abandoned, in order to begin another problem. If there is time at the end, the unfinished problem can always be returned to and completed.

Read the instructions very carefully - twice - so that unpleasant surprises won't follow during or after the exam has ended.

When writing the exam, pretend that the situation is actually simply the completion of homework within a library, or at home. This will assist in forming a relaxed atmosphere, and will allow the brain extra focus for the complex thinking function.

Begin the exam with all of the questions with which the most confidence is felt. This will build the confidence level regarding the entire exam and will begin a quality momentum. This will also create encouragement for trying the problems where uncertainty resides.

Going with the "gut instinct" is always the way to go when solving a problem. Second guessing should be avoided at all costs. Have confidence in the ability to do well.

For essay questions, create an outline in advance that will keep the mind organized and make certain that all of the points are remembered. For multiple choice, read every answer, even if the correct one has been spotted - a better one may exist.

Continue at a pace that is reasonable and not rushed, in order to be able to work carefully. Provide enough time to go over the answers at the end, to check for small errors that can be corrected.

Should a feeling of panic begin, breathe deeply, and think of the feeling of the body releasing sand through its pores. Visualize a calm, peaceful place, and include all of the sights, sounds and sensations of this image. Continue the deep breathing, and take a few minutes to continue this with closed eyes. When all is well again, return to the test.

If a "blanking" occurs for a certain question, skip it and move on to the next question. There will be time to return to the other question later. Get everything done that can be done, first, to guarantee all the grades that can be compiled, and to build all of the confidence possible. Then return to the weaker questions to build the marks from there.

Remember, one's own reality can be created, so as long as the belief is there, success will follow. And remember: anxiety can happen later, right now, there's an exam to be written!

After the examination is complete, whether there is a feeling for a good grade or a bad grade, don't dwell on the exam, and be certain to follow through on the reward that was promised...and enjoy it! Don't dwell on any mistakes that have been made, as there is nothing that can be done at this point anyway.

Additionally, don't begin to study for the next test right away. Do something relaxing for a while, and let the mind relax and prepare itself to begin absorbing information again.

From the results of the exam - both the grade and the entire experience, be certain to learn from what has gone on. Perfect studying habits and work some more on confidence in order to make the next examination experience even better than the last one.

Learn to avoid places where openings occurred for laziness, procrastination and day dreaming.

Use the time between this exam and the next one to better learn to relax, even learning to relax on cue, so that any anxiety can be controlled during the next exam. Learn how to relax the body. Slouch in your chair if that helps. Tighten and then relax all of the different muscle groups, one group at a time, beginning with the feet and then working all the way up to the neck and face. This will ultimately relax the muscles more than they were to begin with. Learn how to breathe deeply and comfortably, and focus on this breathing going in and out as a relaxing thought. With every exhale, repeat the word "relax."

As common as test anxiety is, it is very possible to overcome it. Make yourself one of the test-takers who overcome this frustrating hindrance.

Additional Bonus Material

Due to our efforts to try to keep this book to a manageable length, we've created a link that will give you access to all of your additional bonus material.

Please visit http://www.mometrix.com/bonus948/cphrm to access the information.